Sensual Massage
and Shame

Alaric James Northcott

ISBN: 9798301916731

DEDICATION

To those who seek connections
with themselves, with others, and with the world around
them.
May this book inspire you to embrace the beauty of
vulnerability,
the power of self-awareness, and the courage to rediscover
intimacy in all its forms.
It is for the dreamers, the healers, the explorers of the soul.
And most of all, for you—
who dared to turn the page and begin this journey.
With gratitude and love,
Alaric James Northcott

CONTENTS

ACKNOWLEDGMENTS

This book would not have been possible without many remarkable individuals' support, guidance, and inspiration. To my family and friends, your unwavering encouragement has been the foundation of this journey. Thank you for believing in me, even when I doubt myself. Your love and patience kept me grounded and motivated.
To Mobis Jr, your insights, feedback, and honest conversations helped shape the vision of this book. Your contributions have been invaluable, and I am endlessly grateful for your wisdom and generosity.
To my readers, thank you for choosing to embark on this journey with me. Your curiosity and openness inspire me to continue exploring and sharing.
This book reflects the many voices, lessons, and experiences that have shaped me. Thank you to all who have walked alongside me on this path.
With heartfelt gratitude,

Sensual Massage and Shame:

Exploring Connection, Healing, and Liberation

Sensual massage holds a unique and profound place in the realm of human connection, intimacy, and healing. While it is often associated with pleasure, its depth goes far beyond mere physical gratification. Sensual massage has the potential to heal emotional wounds, deepen intimate bonds, and offer a safe space for self-discovery. Yet, it is often shrouded in societal shame, stigma, and misunderstanding. This article delves into the intersection of sensual massage and shame, exploring their dynamics, the origins of shame in this context, and how sensual touch can serve as a pathway to reclaiming one's body, emotions, and sense of self.

Understanding Sensual Massage

What Is Sensual Massage?

Sensual massage is a holistic practice involving intimate and intentional touch to create relaxation, arousal, and heightened sensory awareness. Unlike therapeutic massages, which focus on physical healing and pain relief, sensual massage emphasizes the emotional and psychological aspects of touch. It can involve:

- Awakening erogenous zones.

- Using techniques to enhance relaxation and intimacy.

- Building a connection between partners or fostering self-awareness.

While sensual massage may incorporate sexual elements, its primary focus is not solely sexual gratification. Instead, it is about exploring the body's potential for pleasure and connection while cultivating trust and intimacy.

The Psychological and Emotional Benefits

Sensual massage offers numerous emotional and psychological benefits, such as:

- **Reducing stress and anxiety:** The practice encourages relaxation, slowing down the mind and body.

Sensual massage is more than just a form of relaxation; it is an art that combines gentle touch to bring calm and balance to both the body and the mind. Through deliberate, gentle and soothing techniques, sensual massage helps slow the pace of modern life, allowing the body to release accumulated tension and enter a deep state of relaxation.

This holistic practice significantly impacts emotional well-being, connecting physical touch with each person's spiritual needs. By reducing stress and anxiety levels, sensual massage becomes a valuable tool for restoring inner harmony. The slow pace and attention paid to each gesture create a safe and comforting atmosphere in which the recipient can completely surrender to the present moment.

Moreover, sensual massage is not just a passive experience; it stimulates the release of endorphins and oxytocin— hormones that contribute to increased happiness, reduced pain, and strengthened emotional bonds between partners. It also promotes a greater awareness of one's own body and personal needs, encouraging the practitioner to be present, accept their vulnerabilities, and explore a deep state of relaxation and self-knowledge.

In a world often marked by agitation and external pressures, sensual massage is an invitation to reconnect with yourself and others. It offers not only physical relaxation but also essential spiritual relief.

Enhancing self-esteem: By fostering appreciation for one's body, it combats negative self-image.

Sensual massage is a relaxation practice and a transformative experience that can significantly improve self-esteem. Fostering a deep appreciation for one's body helps combat negative self-image and encourages a healthier relationship with oneself. Through intentional and caring touch, this practice offers an opportunity to reconnect with the body positively and affirmatively.

Sensual massage's gentle strokes, soothing movements, and mindful presence create a safe space for self-acceptance. It invites individuals to move beyond societal pressures and unrealistic standards, focusing instead on their physical form's inherent beauty and worth. As the body is nurtured and honoured, shame or insecurity often gives way to a profound sense of confidence and self-worth.

Moreover, receiving or giving a sensual massage emphasizes mindfulness and being present in the moment. This attentiveness helps individuals acknowledge and celebrate their body's unique characteristics rather than criticize perceived flaws. Over time, this practice can shift negative thought patterns, replacing them with a more compassionate and appreciative outlook.

Sensual massage can become a powerful tool for boosting self-esteem by reinforcing a sense of worthiness and care. It encourages individuals to embrace their bodies as they are, fostering a holistic sense of well-being that extends beyond the physical into emotional and psychological realms.

Healing trauma: Safe, consensual touch can help individuals reclaim their bodies after experiencing physical or emotional harm.

Sensual massage can be a deeply restorative practice for individuals seeking to heal from physical or emotional trauma. Safe, consensual touch creates an environment of trust and care, helping individuals reclaim their bodies and rebuild a positive relationship with themselves. This process fosters a sense of safety and control, essential components for recovery from trauma.

Trauma often disrupts the connection between mind and body, leading to feelings of disassociation, fear, or discomfort with physical touch. Sensual massage, when approached with sensitivity and respect, provides a pathway to restore this connection gently. The slow, intentional movements allow individuals to explore their physical sensations in a secure and nurturing context, promoting a sense of grounding and presence in the moment.

By prioritizing consent and clear communication, sensual massage empowers individuals to set boundaries and voice their needs, helping to rebuild a sense of agency and trust. This emphasis on mutual respect ensures that the experience is healing and empowering, as it reinforces the individual's right to feel safe and in control of their body.

Additionally, sensual massage encourages the release of stored tension and emotional pain held within the body. The therapeutic touch can facilitate the body's natural healing processes, helping to dissolve the physical manifestations of trauma, such as muscle tightness or chronic stress.

Over time, this practice can help individuals replace fear and discomfort with feelings of acceptance, comfort, and even joy in their bodies. It becomes a stepping stone toward reclaiming a sense of wholeness and well-being, allowing individuals to move forward with greater confidence and resilience.

Deepening intimacy: Couples can use sensual massage to strengthen bonds and rebuild trust.

Sensual massage can be a powerful way for couples to deepen intimacy, strengthen emotional bonds, and rebuild trust. The art of intentional, caring touch fosters a safe and nurturing environment where partners can connect on a deeper physical and emotional level.

In relationships, touch is crucial in expressing love, care, and support. Sensual massage takes this further by encouraging both partners to be fully present and attuned to each other's needs. The slow, deliberate movements and shared experience create a sense of vulnerability and openness, essential for fostering intimacy and trust.

As couples engage in this practice, they become more aware of each other's bodies and emotions. Giving and receiving massage becomes a non-verbal communication tool, allowing them to express affection, gratitude, and understanding. This mutual exchange of care helps to break down barriers and strengthen the emotional connection.

Sensual massage also provides a space for couples to prioritize each other, away from the distractions and stresses of daily life. By dedicating time to nurture the relationship, partners reaffirm their commitment and appreciation for one another, rekindling passion and closeness.

Sensual massage can be incredibly healing for relationships that have experienced strain or disconnection. The emphasis on trust and consent enables couples to rebuild emotional safety, while physical intimacy helps to reestablish a sense of partnership and unity.

Over time, this shared practice can enhance physical and emotional intimacy, creating a stronger, more loving bond between partners. It reminds us of the importance of touch and connection in maintaining a healthy and fulfilling relationship.

Despite these benefits, sensual massage Is often clouded by shame due to cultural, societal, and personal factors.

The Origins of Shame in Sensuality

Shame is a deeply ingrained emotion, often tied to societal norms, cultural taboos, and personal experiences. It manifests as a sense of inadequacy, guilt, or fear, particularly in matters of intimacy and pleasure. To understand its impact on sensual massage, it's essential to examine its sources.

1. Cultural and Religious Conditioning

Throughout history, many cultures and religious doctrines have imposed strict moral codes on sexuality and intimacy. Teachings that label sensuality as sinful, immoral, or shameful have left lasting imprints. Sensual massage, which involves intimate touch, often becomes entangled in these beliefs, perpetuating guilt and discomfort.

For example:

- **Religious taboos:** Some religious traditions discourage any form of touch associated with pleasure, framing it as indulgent or impure.

- **Cultural modesty:** Societies with conservative values may stigmatize practices involving nudity or intimate touch, fostering embarrassment.

2. Body Image and Media Influence

Media plays a significant role in shaping societal attitudes toward the body and sensuality. Unrealistic beauty standards and sexualized imagery often lead individuals to feel inadequate or ashamed of their appearance. Sensual massage, which involves vulnerability and body acceptance, can feel threatening to those burdened by body-related shame.

3. Trauma and Negative Experiences

For individuals who have experienced abuse, assault, or other forms of trauma, the connection between touch and safety may be fractured. Sensual massage, even when consensual, can trigger feelings of vulnerability, fear, or shame. These reactions are often rooted in past experiences where boundaries were violated.

4. Fear of Judgment and Vulnerability

Shame often stems from the fear of being judged or misunderstood. Sensual massage requires openness and vulnerability, which can be intimidating. Individuals may worry about being perceived as immoral, unattractive, or overly indulgent.

How Sensual Massage Challenges and Heals Shame

Sensual massage has the potential to dismantle shame and replace it with empowerment, confidence, and self-love. Through its focus on intentional touch, consent, and connection, it offers a path to healing and liberation.

1. Reclaiming the Body

Shame often creates a disconnect between individuals and their bodies, fostering feelings of alienation or disdain. Sensual massage helps bridge this gap by encouraging individuals to experience their bodies in a nurturing and non-judgmental way. It fosters:

- **Awareness:** Sensual massage invites participants to focus on their body's sensations, helping them reconnect with physical and emotional responses.

  Sensual massage is a practice that encourages participants to reconnect with their physical and emotional selves by focusing on the body's sensations. This heightened awareness fosters a deeper understanding of one's responses, promoting self-discovery and inner harmony.

  In the fast-paced rhythm of modern life, many individuals become disconnected from their bodies, losing touch with the subtle signals and sensations that reflect physical and emotional well-being. Sensual massage offers a grounding experience, inviting participants to slow down and attune to the present moment. The gentle, deliberate touch helps individuals become more aware of their body's needs, desires, and areas of tension.

As the practice unfolds, participants are encouraged to observe and embrace their physical sensations without judgment. This mindfulness cultivates a deeper connection with the body, allowing a greater understanding of how emotions manifest physically. Over time, this awareness can improve emotional regulation and balance.

Sensual massage also creates a safe space for exploring and honouring the body's responses, whether related to relaxation, pleasure, or emotional release. This exploration fosters self-acceptance and helps individuals develop a more compassionate relationship with themselves.

Sensual massage bridges the gap between physical and emotional awareness, empowering participants to reconnect with their inner selves. It becomes a transformative practice, enhancing self-awareness and overall well-being.

- **Acceptance:** By celebrating the body's capacity for pleasure, sensual massage encourages self-acceptance and appreciation.

Sensual massage is a beautiful way to foster self-acceptance by celebrating the body's capacity for pleasure and connection. It offers a nurturing experience encouraging individuals to appreciate and honour their bodies, promoting a sense of self-worth and acceptance.

In a world often dominated by unrealistic beauty standards and self-criticism, sensual massage provides an opportunity to shift focus from perceived imperfections to the body's incredible ability to feel, heal, and connect. The gentle, intentional touch serves as a reminder of the body's inherent value and beauty, helping to cultivate a positive self-image.

Sensual massage helps individuals learn to embrace their physical selves with kindness and compassion. The practice invites them to explore their bodies without judgment, focusing instead on the sensations, pleasure, and relaxation of mindful touch. This deepened awareness fosters a sense of gratitude for the body's resilience and capabilities.

The experience of sensual massage also promotes mindfulness, encouraging individuals to be fully present in their bodies and the moment. This presence helps to quiet negative self-talk and replace it with an appreciation for the body's unique qualities and strengths.

Over time, the practice of sensual massage can transform one's relationship with one's body, shifting it from one of criticism to one of acceptance and celebration. It becomes a powerful tool for cultivating self-love and appreciating the body as a source of joy and well-being.

For many, this process is transformative, especially for those who have experienced shame related to body image or past trauma.

2. Establishing Safe and Consensual Boundaries

Consent is a cornerstone of sensual massage. Practitioners and participants must communicate openly about their comfort levels, boundaries, and intentions. This focus on mutual respect helps individuals feel safe and respected, counteracting feelings of shame or fear.

Key elements include:

- Clear communication before and during the session.

- Respecting boundaries without judgment.

- Creating a space of mutual trust and understanding.

3. Promoting Emotional Release

The body often holds onto emotional pain, particularly when it is tied to shame or trauma. Sensual massage can help release these pent-up emotions by creating a safe space for expression. Tears, laughter, or verbal acknowledgments are common during or after a session, signalling the release of suppressed feelings.

4. Encouraging Vulnerability and Trust

Shame thrives in secrecy and isolation. Sensual massage challenges this by encouraging vulnerability in a controlled and supportive environment. Participants learn that being open about their desires, fears, and boundaries is not only acceptable but also necessary for genuine connection.

Practical Steps to Overcome Shame Through Sensual Massage

Overcoming shame and embracing sensual massage as a tool for healing requires intentional effort and a supportive environment. Here are practical steps to facilitate this journey:

1. Begin with Self-Exploration

Self-massage is an excellent starting point for those who feel uncomfortable or ashamed. It allows individuals to explore their bodies in a private, judgment-free setting. Incorporating soothing elements such as scented oils, calming music, or candles can enhance the experience.

2. Seek Professional Guidance

For individuals struggling with significant shame or trauma, working with a certified sensual massage therapist or somatic healer can be invaluable. These professionals are trained to navigate the emotional complexities that may arise and provide a safe and supportive environment.

3. Communicate Openly with Partners

If engaging in sensual massage with a partner, communication is key. Discuss fears, boundaries, and expectations openly to build trust and reduce the fear of judgment.

4. Create a Safe and Inviting Environment

The setting plays a crucial role in making sensual massage a positive experience. A comfortable, warm, and private space with calming elements (e.g., dim lighting, soft fabrics, or relaxing aromas) can help participants feel at ease.

5. Incorporate Mindfulness Practices

Mindfulness encourages individuals to focus on the present moment without judgment. By pairing sensual massage with deep breathing or meditation, participants can heighten their awareness of physical sensations and reduce feelings of shame or anxiety.

Real-Life Transformations: Stories of Healing

Anna's Journey

Anna, a survivor of sexual trauma, had long struggled with intimacy. Through guided sensual massage therapy, she gradually learned to associate touch with safety and care. Over time, the practice helped her rebuild trust in herself and her relationships, transforming her fear of vulnerability into empowerment.

Mark and Lisa's Bond

After years of emotional distance, Mark and Lisa turned to sensual massage to rekindle their intimacy. By prioritizing touch and communication, they rediscovered their connection and deepened their relationship.

Raj's Self-Acceptance

Raj, who struggled with body-image issues, began practicing self-massage to confront his insecurities. Over time, he developed a newfound appreciation for his body's resilience and capabilities, replacing shame with self-confidence.

Addressing Stigma and Promoting Understanding

Sensual massage remains misunderstood and stigmatized due to its association with sexuality. Breaking down these barriers requires advocacy, education, and open dialogue.

1. Educating the Public

Workshops, articles, and social media platforms can highlight the therapeutic and emotional benefits of sensual massage, dispelling myths and misconceptions.

2. Normalizing Vulnerability

By sharing personal stories of healing and transformation, individuals can challenge societal taboos and demonstrate the profound impact of sensual massage.

3. Encouraging Inclusivity

Sensual massage should be presented as a practice for everyone, regardless of gender, age, or relationship status. This inclusivity helps reduce stigma and fosters a sense of belonging.

Conclusion

Sensual massage offers a powerful pathway to connection, healing, and liberation. By confronting shame and embracing intentional touch, individuals can reclaim their sense of self, build deeper connections with others, and foster a more positive relationship with their bodies.

Though societal shame and misunderstanding remain significant barriers, sensual massage has the potential to transform lives by promoting trust, acceptance, and emotional freedom. It is a profound reminder that the body is not a source of shame but a vessel for connection, pleasure, and healing. By creating safe spaces for vulnerability and celebration, we can move closer to a world where sensuality is embraced as a natural and empowering part of the human experience.

Is It Good to Be Ashamed, or Does Shame Deprive You of Freedom?

Shame is one of the most complex emotions in the human experience, touching on self-perception, societal norms, and personal growth. It arises when individuals feel they have failed to meet a standard—whether it's their own or one imposed by others. At its best, shame can serve as a moral compass, guiding behaviour and fostering accountability. However, when left unchecked, shame can become oppressive, leading to feelings of inadequacy, isolation, and the loss of freedom.

This article explores the dual nature of shame, examining when it can be constructive and when it becomes a barrier to emotional and psychological freedom. By understanding the nuances of shame, individuals can navigate its effects more effectively and foster a healthier relationship with themselves and others.

Understanding Shame: A Dual Perspective

Shame is often conflated with guilt, but the two emotions are distinct. While guilt focuses on specific actions ("I did something bad"), shame targets the self ("I am bad"). This self-directed nature makes shame uniquely powerful, as it can deeply affect an individual's identity and sense of worth.

The Role of Shame in Human Evolution

From an evolutionary perspective, shame likely developed as a social emotion to promote group cohesion and survival. Early human communities relied on cooperation, and shame acted as a deterrent against behaviour's that could jeopardize the group's well-being. Feeling ashamed for violating social norms encouraged individuals to conform, fostering harmony and mutual trust.

However, the social utility of shame doesn't always translate into positive outcomes. In modern societies, where norms are varied and often conflicting, shame can become a source of emotional distress rather than a constructive guide.

When Shame Is Beneficial

Despite its negative connotations, shame can serve important purposes in personal and social contexts. When experienced in moderation and processed constructively, shame can lead to growth, empathy, and ethical behaviour.

1. Shame as a Moral Compass

Shame can act as an internal alarm system, signalling when one's actions have deviated from personal or societal values. For instance:

- Feeling ashamed after lying or hurting someone can prompt reflection and encourage corrective actions.

- Recognizing shame can strengthen accountability, fostering a commitment to integrity and honesty.

In this context, shame helps individuals align their behaviour with their values, contributing to personal growth and stronger relationships.

2. Building Empathy and Compassion

Experiencing shame can increase empathy, as it creates an understanding of the emotional pain caused by certain actions. This awareness can:

- Foster compassion for others who experience similar struggles.

- Strengthen interpersonal connections by promoting sensitivity to others' feelings.

For example, someone who has felt ashamed of their mistakes may be more forgiving of others, creating a culture of mutual support and understanding.

3. Motivation for Self-Improvement

Shame, when channelled constructively, can inspire self-improvement. It highlights areas where growth is needed, pushing individuals to:

- Develop new skills or habits.

- Address harmful behaviour's.

- Seek support or therapy to overcome personal challenges.

In this way, shame becomes a catalyst for positive change, helping individuals achieve their potential.

When Shame Becomes Harmful

While shame has the potential to guide and motivate, it often crosses the line into harmful territory. When shame is excessive, chronic, or tied to an individual's identity rather than their actions, it can be profoundly damaging.

1. Erosion of Self-Worth

When shame becomes internalized, it shifts from focusing on behaviour ("I did something wrong") to attacking the self ("I am fundamentally flawed"). This erosion of self-worth can lead to:

- **Low self-esteem:** Persistent feelings of inadequacy or unworthiness.

- **Self-sabotage:** Believing one is undeserving of success or happiness.

- **Negative self-talk:** A constant inner dialogue of criticism and self-judgment.

This type of shame is particularly common among individuals who have experienced trauma, abuse, or rejection.

2. Social Isolation

Shame often leads individuals to withdraw from others out of fear of judgment or rejection. This isolation can:

- Create a sense of loneliness and disconnection.

- Prevent individuals from seeking support or sharing their experiences.

- Exacerbate feelings of unworthiness and alienation.

Ironically, the more someone isolates themselves due to shame, the harder it becomes to break the cycle of self-blame and fear.

3. Suppression of Authenticity

Shame can pressure individuals to conform to societal norms, even when those norms conflict with their true selves. For example:

- Someone may suppress their sexual orientation, beliefs, or passions to avoid societal judgment.

- They may feel compelled to hide vulnerabilities or emotions, creating a facade of perfection.

This suppression of authenticity deprives individuals of the freedom to express themselves fully and live in alignment with their values.

4. Impact on Mental Health

Chronic shame is a significant risk factor for mental health issues, including:

- **Depression:** A pervasive sense of hopelessness and worthlessness.

- **Anxiety:** Fear of judgment or failure leading to constant vigilance and stress.

- **Addiction:** Using substances or behaviours to numb the pain of shame.

In extreme cases, shame can lead to suicidal thoughts, as individuals feel trapped in a cycle of self-loathing.

Balancing Shame: Finding Freedom Through Awareness

The key to navigating shame lies in distinguishing between its constructive and destructive forms. By developing self-awareness and adopting healthy coping strategies, individuals can use shame as a tool for growth while minimizing its harmful effects.

1. Recognize and Name Shame

The first step in addressing shame is to identify when it is present. Naming the emotion helps create distance from it, making it easier to analyse and manage. Questions to ask Include:

- What triggered this feeling of shame?

- Is the shame tied to my actions, or is it targeting my sense of self?

- Does this shame align with my personal values, or is it imposed by external expectations?

2. Reframe Shame as an Opportunity

Rather than viewing shame as purely negative, individuals can reframe it as a learning experience. For example:

- If shame arises from a mistake, focus on what can be done to make amends or improve in the future.

- If shame is tied to societal judgment, question whether those norms truly align with one's values.

Reframing shame shifts the focus from self-punishment to self-growth.

3. Cultivate Self-Compassion

Self-compassion is a powerful antidote to shame. By treating oneself with kindness and understanding, individuals can:

- Counteract negative self-talk with affirmations of worth and value.

- Recognize that mistakes and imperfections are part of the human experience.

- Foster resilience in the face of setbacks or criticism.

Practices like mindfulness, journaling, or therapy can help build self-compassion over time.

4. Seek Connection

Shame often thrives in secrecy and isolation. Sharing experiences with trusted friends, family, or support groups can help dismantle the power of shame. These connections remind individuals that:

- They are not alone in their struggles.

- Vulnerability can strengthen relationships rather than weaken them.

- Others have likely faced similar challenges and can offer guidance or empathy.

Shame and Freedom: The Complex Relationship

To answer the question, "Is it good to be ashamed, or does shame deprive you of freedom?" one must consider the context and intensity of the emotion.

When Shame Guides Freedom

In its constructive form, shame can enhance freedom by:

- Encouraging ethical behaviour that aligns with personal and societal values.

- Motivating individuals to grow and improve, leading to greater self-confidence and autonomy.

- Strengthening relationships through accountability and empathy.

In these cases, shame serves as a guide, helping individuals navigate their choices with integrity and self-awareness.

When Shame Restricts Freedom

Conversely, shame can deprive individuals of freedom when it:

- Becomes internalized, leading to self-doubt and feelings of unworthiness.

- Promotes conformity to harmful or oppressive societal norms.

- Suppresses authenticity, preventing individuals from living in alignment with their true selves.

In these instances, shame acts as a barrier, limiting one's ability to experience joy, connection, and self-expression.

Moving Toward Freedom

To move beyond the restrictive effects of shame, individuals can adopt practices that promote self-awareness, acceptance, and liberation. These include:

- **Challenging societal norms:** Questioning whether external expectations align with personal values.

- **Practicing forgiveness:** Letting go of past mistakes and recognizing that they do not define one's worth.

- **Embracing vulnerability:** Viewing openness and authenticity as strengths rather than weaknesses.

Ultimately, freedom comes from understanding that shame is not an inherent flaw but a signal—one that can guide behaviour or highlight areas for growth when approached with compassion and mindfulness.

Conclusion

Shame is neither inherently good nor bad; its impact depends on how it is experienced and processed. When used constructively, shame can guide ethical behaviour, foster empathy, and inspire self-improvement. However, when it becomes internalized or excessive, shame can erode self-worth, suppress authenticity, and deprive individuals of emotional and psychological freedom.

By recognizing the dual nature of shame and adopting strategies to navigate it effectively, individuals can transform this complex emotion into a source of growth rather than a barrier. In doing so, they reclaim their freedom to live authentically, connect deeply, and embrace their inherent worth.

How Should a Normal Person React to a Sensual Massage from a Shame Perspective?

Sensual massage is a powerful and intimate practice that fosters relaxation, connection, and healing. Yet, for many, it is accompanied by complex emotional reactions, especially feelings of shame. Shame arises from a perceived violation of societal norms, personal boundaries, or internalized values, and it can heavily influence how a person reacts to a sensual massage.

This article explores how a "normal" person—that is, someone navigating common societal, cultural, and personal influences—might react to a sensual massage through the lens of shame. It will discuss the origins of these shame-related reactions, strategies for navigating them, and ways to foster a healthier, more empowering perspective on sensual massage.

Understanding the Role of Shame in Sensual Massage

What Is Shame?

Shame is an emotion that targets the self, creating feelings of inadequacy, guilt, or embarrassment. Unlike guilt, which is tied to specific actions, shame makes a person feel flawed or unworthy. This internalized belief can influence how people perceive their bodies, their actions, and their interactions with others.

In the context of sensual massage, shame may arise due to:

- Societal taboos about touch and intimacy.

- Personal insecurities about the body or its functions.

- Internalized cultural or religious teachings about morality and propriety.

- Fear of judgment or misinterpretation of the intent behind receiving or giving sensual touch.

Why Shame Is Common During Sensual Massage

Sensual massage inherently involves vulnerability. It often includes elements such as physical nudity, close proximity to another person, and the exploration of sensation and pleasure. These factors can trigger deeply rooted feelings of discomfort or fear of judgment. Many people are conditioned to view sensuality as private or even shameful, which can lead to conflicting emotions during the experience.

A Spectrum of Reactions to Sensual Massage

A person's reaction to a sensual massage depends on their cultural background, personal history, and emotional state. Reactions can range from curiosity and enjoyment to discomfort or even guilt. Let's explore these responses in detail:

1. Curiosity and Openness

Some individuals approach sensual massage with curiosity, viewing it as an opportunity for relaxation, healing, or self-exploration. They may:

- Feel intrigued by the idea of experiencing intentional touch.

- Be open to exploring their emotions and physical sensations without judgment.

- Recognize the potential therapeutic and emotional benefits of the practice.

For these individuals, shame is less likely to dominate their experience. They may have already worked to dismantle internalized taboos or view sensuality as a natural and empowering aspect of life.

2. Embarrassment or Awkwardness

For many, the initial reaction to a sensual massage is a mix of embarrassment and awkwardness. These feelings often stem from:

- Unfamiliarity with the practice.

- Worry about how their body will be perceived.

- Fear of unintentionally expressing or experiencing arousal.

This reaction is common and can be addressed through clear communication and a supportive environment.

3. Discomfort and Shame

Some individuals feel deeply uncomfortable or ashamed during a sensual massage. These feelings may manifest as:

- Self-consciousness about their appearance, weight, or perceived imperfections.

- Fear of being judged or misunderstood by the massage practitioner or partner.

- Internal conflict between enjoying the sensations and feeling guilty about them.

In these cases, shame often acts as a barrier to fully experiencing the benefits of the massage.

4. Emotional Overwhelm

Sensual massage can also evoke strong emotional responses, such as crying, laughter, or feelings of release. These reactions are natural and often indicate the release of stored emotions. However, they can be unsettling if the individual is unprepared or unsure how to interpret them.

Navigating Shame During a Sensual Massage

For those who experience shame during a sensual massage, it's important to recognize that these feelings are valid but not insurmountable. With self-awareness and the right strategies, individuals can work through their shame and embrace the experience more fully.

1. Reflect on the Source of Shame

Understanding why shame arises is the first step in addressing it. Common sources include:

- **Cultural Conditioning:** Consider whether societal norms or religious teachings have shaped your views on touch and sensuality.

- **Personal Insecurities:** Reflect on whether shame stems from self-consciousness about your body or fears of vulnerability.

- **Past Experiences:** Acknowledge whether past trauma or negative touch has influenced your reaction.

Naming the source of shame helps to demystify it and provides a foundation for growth.

2. Practice Self-Compassion

Self-compassion is a powerful antidote to shame. By treating yourself with kindness and understanding, you can create a safe internal environment for exploring your feelings. Try:

- **Affirmations:** Repeat phrases like, "My body is worthy of care and respect," or "It's okay to feel vulnerable."

- **Mindfulness:** Focus on the present moment rather than getting caught up in self-criticism or judgment.

- **Forgiveness:** Let go of guilt or self-blame for feeling conflicted or emotional.

3. Communicate Your Feelings

If you're receiving a sensual massage from a partner or professional, open communication is essential. Share your concerns, boundaries, and emotions to create a more supportive experience. For example:

- Let your partner or therapist know if you feel self-conscious or need reassurance.

- Discuss any areas of your body that feel particularly sensitive or vulnerable.

- Ask for pauses or adjustments if you start to feel overwhelmed.

4. Focus on Consent and Boundaries

Establishing clear boundaries can help mitigate feelings of shame or discomfort. Before the massage, discuss:

- **What feels safe and comfortable:** Be specific about areas of the body that are okay to touch.

- **Intentions for the massage:** Frame the experience as a practice of relaxation and connection, not a performance or obligation.

- **Signals for communication:** Agree on nonverbal cues, such as raising a hand, to signal the need for a break.

Having these agreements in place reinforces your sense of agency and control.

Transforming Shame Into Empowerment

By addressing shame head-on, individuals can transform it into a source of growth and empowerment. Sensual massage becomes not just a physical practice but a journey toward self-acceptance and liberation.

1. Embrace Vulnerability

Sensual massage inherently requires a degree of vulnerability, but this openness can be a source of strength. Vulnerability allows you to:

- Build deeper connections with others.

- Acknowledge and honour your emotional needs.

- Experience intimacy and trust in new ways.

Reframing vulnerability as a positive quality can help dissolve shame and foster greater self-confidence.

2. Reframe Sensuality

Many people associate sensuality with shame due to societal taboos or misunderstandings. Reframing sensuality as a natural and empowering aspect of life can shift this perspective. Consider:

- Viewing sensual massage as an act of self-care, not indulgence.

- Recognizing the body as a vessel for connection, healing, and pleasure.

- Celebrating the unique beauty and capabilities of your body.

3. Focus on the Benefits

Rather than dwelling on feelings of shame, redirect your attention to the positive aspects of the experience. Sensual massage offers:

- Physical relaxation and stress relief.

- Enhanced mindfulness and body awareness.

- Emotional release and healing.

By focusing on these benefits, you can cultivate gratitude and reduce the power of shame.

The Role of Societal Change

While personal strategies are crucial, addressing the societal roots of shame can create a more supportive environment for sensual massage. Advocating for open dialogue, education, and inclusivity can help normalize this practice and reduce stigma.

1. Educate Others

Raising awareness about the therapeutic and emotional benefits of sensual massage can challenge misconceptions and promote understanding. Share resources, articles, or personal experiences to spark conversation.

2. Advocate for Inclusivity

Sensual massage is for everyone, regardless of gender, age, or relationship status. Highlighting diverse perspectives can break down stereotypes and make the practice more accessible.

3. Promote Body Positivity

Encouraging body acceptance and celebrating diverse forms of beauty can counteract the shame many people feel about their appearance. This cultural shift can create a more supportive environment for practices like sensual massage.

Conclusion

A normal person's reaction to a sensual massage, when viewed through the lens of shame, is shaped by societal conditioning, personal insecurities, and individual experiences. While feelings of shame are natural, they do not have to dominate the experience. By reflecting on the sources of shame, practicing self-compassion, communicating openly, and embracing vulnerability, individuals can transform sensual massage into a powerful tool for self-acceptance and connection.

As society becomes more open to discussions about touch, intimacy, and emotional healing, sensual massage can be reframed as a practice of empowerment rather than a source of shame. Through education, advocacy, and inclusivity, we can create a culture where individuals feel free to explore and celebrate their bodies without fear or judgment.

Understanding Sensual Massage: A Holistic Perspective

Sensual massage is an ancient and profoundly healing practice that transcends physical touch, delving into the realms of emotional connection, self-awareness, and intimacy. While it is often associated with arousal and pleasure, its essence goes far beyond the mere stimulation of erogenous zones. Sensual massage is a holistic practice that honours the connection between the body and mind, offering benefits that include physical relaxation, emotional release, and intimacy enhancement.

Despite these positive aspects, sensual massage is often misunderstood, and its profound benefits are obscured by cultural taboos and misconceptions about sexuality. This article explores the essence of sensual massage, its benefits, techniques, and its place in a modern context as a practice of connection and healing.

The Fundamentals of Sensual Massage

What Is Sensual Massage?

At its core, sensual massage is a form of intentional touch designed to relax the body, awaken sensory awareness, and cultivate a deeper connection with oneself or a partner. The practice often involves:

- Long, flowing strokes.

- Use of oils, scents, and calming music to stimulate the senses.

- Techniques that may include light pressure, kneading, or gentle tapping.

It may also focus on areas of the body that hold tension, including the back, shoulders, and feet, while incorporating the stimulation of erogenous zones when appropriate. However, sensual massage is not inherently sexual; it prioritizes connection, relaxation, and self-awareness over physical gratification.

A Brief History

The origins of sensual massage can be traced to ancient traditions like:

- **Ayurveda:** An Indian practice that incorporates therapeutic massage with oils to balance the body's energies.

- **Tantra:** A spiritual practice that often includes intimate touch to awaken and harmonize life energy.

- **Traditional Chinese Medicine (TCM):** Where massage is used to unblock energy pathways, or meridians, in the body.

These traditions emphasize the role of touch as a conduit for healing, connection, and spiritual growth, setting the stage for modern interpretations of sensual massage.

The Holistic Benefits of Sensual Massage

Sensual massage provides a wealth of physical, emotional, and relational benefits. Its holistic nature makes it a transformative practice for individuals and couples alike.

1. Physical Relaxation

Touch is a powerful tool for relieving tension and soothing the body. Sensual massage offers:

- **Muscle relaxation:** Techniques like kneading and stroking help release knots and tightness.

- **Improved circulation:** The use of long strokes enhances blood flow, promoting oxygenation and detoxification of the body.

- **Nervous system regulation:** Gentle, rhythmic touch activates the parasympathetic nervous system, calming the body and reducing stress.

2. Emotional Release

The emotional benefits of sensual massage are often overlooked but are deeply impactful:

- **Stress relief:** By creating a safe and soothing environment, sensual massage helps reduce cortisol levels, promoting a sense of calm.

- **Emotional connection:** Touch can unlock buried emotions, allowing individuals to confront and release pent-up feelings of grief, anger, or sadness.

- **Self-awareness:** Sensual massage encourages mindfulness, fostering a deeper understanding of one's emotional state.

3. Intimacy Enhancement

For couples, sensual massage is a powerful way to deepen their connection:

- **Building trust:** The act of giving and receiving touch requires vulnerability and trust, strengthening emotional bonds.

- **Improved communication:** Couples often find that the practice helps them express desires, boundaries, and affection more openly.

- **Rekindling passion:** By focusing on physical and emotional connection, sensual massage can reignite intimacy and closeness.

The Sensory Experience of Sensual Massage

Sensual massage is a multisensory experience that engages sight, sound, touch, and smell. Each element plays a role in creating a harmonious and transformative practice.

1. Touch: The Primary Medium

Touch is the foundation of sensual massage, providing physical and emotional comfort. The techniques used range from light brushing to firm pressure, depending on the desired outcome. Practitioners may focus on:

- **Erogenous zones** for arousal and intimacy.

- **Tension areas** like the shoulders, neck, or lower back for relaxation.

2. Scent: Enhancing the Atmosphere

Aromatherapy oils such as lavender, rose, or sandalwood are often incorporated to heighten relaxation and sensory pleasure. Scents can evoke specific emotional states, such as calmness or passion.

3. Sound: Setting the Tone

Music plays an essential role in sensual massage, helping to create an environment conducive to relaxation. Soft instrumental tracks or nature sounds are common choices to encourage mindfulness and immersion.

4. Sight: Creating Comfort

Lighting and decor also impact the sensual massage experience. Dim lighting, candles, or soft fabrics can make the space feel more inviting and safer.

Techniques for Sensual Massage

Sensual massage techniques vary depending on the intent—whether to relax, arouse, or create intimacy. Below are some common approaches:

1. Effleurage

Effleurage involves long, gliding strokes using the palms. This technique is ideal for warming up the muscles and increasing circulation. It is particularly soothing for the back, arms, and legs.

2. Feather Touch

A light, gentle touch with the fingertips or feathers can heighten sensitivity and arousal. This technique is best used on erogenous zones or areas with delicate skin.

3. Kneading

Kneading involves applying firm pressure with the hands to work out muscle tension. It is often used on the shoulders, thighs, or feet.

4. Circular Motions

Circular motions with the palms or fingertips can be used to massage joints or smaller muscle groups, promoting relaxation and flexibility.

Overcoming Misconceptions About Sensual Massage

Despite its many benefits, sensual massage is often misunderstood due to societal taboos and cultural misconceptions.

1. The Association with Sexuality

Sensual massage is often conflated with sexual activity, leading to stigma. While it may incorporate elements of intimacy, its primary purpose is to connect the mind and body, not to achieve sexual gratification.

2. The Fear of Vulnerability

Many people shy away from sensual massage due to the vulnerability it requires. Addressing this fear involves:

- **Educating oneself:** Understanding the therapeutic and emotional benefits of the practice.

- **Communicating openly:** Discussing boundaries and expectations with a partner or practitioner.

3. Body Image Concerns

Self-consciousness about one's body can hinder the ability to fully experience sensual massage. Practices such as self-massage or mindfulness can help individuals embrace their bodies and feel more comfortable with touch.

Incorporating Sensual Massage into Daily Life

Sensual massage does not have to be reserved for special occasions; it can be integrated into daily routines to promote relaxation and connection.

1. Self-Massage

Self-massage is a great way to experience the benefits of sensual touch without the need for a partner. Techniques include:

- Using oils to massage the arms, legs, or feet.

- Applying gentle pressure to the temples to relieve stress.

- Practicing mindfulness to focus on sensations and emotions.

2. Partner Massage

Couples can use sensual massage to nurture their relationship. Setting aside time for intentional touch fosters intimacy and strengthens bonds. Key tips include:

- **Creating a ritual:** Dedicate a specific time and space for the practice.

- **Communicating needs:** Share preferences and boundaries to ensure comfort and trust.

Sensual Massage in a Professional Context

For those seeking guided experiences, professional practitioners can provide therapeutic sensual massages tailored to individual needs. When choosing a professional:

- Ensure they are certified and reputable.

- Discuss goals and boundaries beforehand.

- Choose a practitioner who creates a safe and respectful environment.

The Future of Sensual Massage

As society evolves, the perception of sensual massage is slowly shifting. Increasing awareness of its holistic benefits is paving the way for greater acceptance. Key developments include:

- **Integration into wellness programs:** Sensual massage is being recognized as a valuable component of mental health and wellness practices.

- **Educational initiatives:** Workshops and resources are helping to demystify the practice and reduce stigma.

- **Inclusivity:** Sensual massage is becoming more accessible to people of all genders, ages, and relationship statuses.

Conclusion

Sensual massage is a profound and multifaceted practice that offers numerous physical, emotional, and relational benefits. By focusing on intentional touch, sensory engagement, and connection, it serves as a gateway to relaxation, self-awareness, and intimacy. Despite cultural misconceptions and taboos, sensual massage holds immense potential as a holistic tool for healing and growth.

As more individuals embrace its transformative power, sensual massage can help break down barriers of shame and misunderstanding, paving the way for a deeper connection with oneself and others. Whether practiced solo, with a partner, or under professional guidance, sensual massage is a journey into the art of touch and the beauty of human connection.

The Role of Shame in the Human Experience

Shame is one of the most deeply ingrained and complex emotions in the human experience. Unlike guilt, which is linked to specific actions and behaviours, shame targets the self, creating a pervasive sense of unworthiness or inadequacy. It arises from the perception of having violated social norms, personal values, or cultural expectations. This powerful emotion shapes how individuals see themselves, their relationships with others, and their sense of belonging in the world.

In the context of sensuality and practices like sensual massage, shame often emerges due to societal messages about the body, pleasure, and intimacy. This article explores the multifaceted role of shame in human life, with a focus on its sources, manifestations, and the ways it impacts sensuality, touch, and healing.

Understanding Shame: A Core Human Emotion

The Nature of Shame

Shame can be defined as the emotional response to the belief that one is fundamentally flawed, bad, or unworthy. It is a universal emotion, experienced across all cultures and societies, though its triggers and expressions vary widely. Shame is distinct from guilt in that:

- **Guilt** relates to actions ("I did something wrong").

- **Shame** targets the self ("I am wrong").

This self-directed nature of shame makes it uniquely powerful and potentially damaging. While guilt can motivate corrective action, shame often leads to withdrawal, isolation, and self-condemnation.

The Evolutionary Role of Shame

From an evolutionary perspective, shame likely developed as a social emotion to promote group cohesion and cooperation. In early human societies, being ostracized or rejected by the group could mean death. Shame served as a mechanism to regulate behaviour, encouraging individuals to conform to social norms and avoid actions that could jeopardize their inclusion in the group.

Sources of Shame Related to Sensuality

Sensuality and intimacy are deeply personal aspects of human life that are often intertwined with cultural, societal, and personal influences. Shame related to sensuality frequently arises from the following sources:

1. Cultural and Religious Conditioning

Many cultures and religions impose strict guidelines about physical touch, nudity, and sexual expression. These teachings can create a pervasive sense of fear or guilt surrounding the body and its desires.

Religious Taboos and Morality

Religious doctrines often emphasize modesty, chastity, and control over bodily desires. While these teachings can provide structure and moral guidance, they can also instill shame in individuals who deviate from prescribed norms. Sensual massage, which involves intimate touch and often evokes pleasure, can become entangled with notions of immorality or sinfulness.

For example:

- **Western traditions:** Many Abrahamic religions (Christianity, Islam, Judaism) emphasize purity and often associate physical pleasure with moral failing.

- **Eastern philosophies:** While some traditions like Tantra celebrate sensuality as a spiritual practice, others promote asceticism, viewing bodily desires as distractions from enlightenment.

Cultural Modesty and Gender Roles

Cultural norms about modesty and propriety can exacerbate shame around sensuality. Women are often subjected to strict expectations about their appearance, behaviour, and sexual expression. In many cultures, women who embrace their sensuality risk being labelled as immoral or immodest, fostering internalized shame.

2. Media and Societal Expectations

The media plays a significant role in shaping societal attitudes toward beauty, sexuality, and relationships. It perpetuates unrealistic standards that contribute to feelings of inadequacy and shame.

Unrealistic Beauty Ideals

Media portrayals of the "perfect" body—often young, thin, and flawless—create unattainable standards for most people. These images can lead to body shame, particularly in the context of practices like sensual massage, which involve vulnerability and self-acceptance. Individuals who do not meet these ideals may feel unworthy of being touched or appreciated.

Sexual Objectification

Media often sexualizes bodies, reducing them to objects of desire rather than honouring their intrinsic value. This commodification can lead individuals to feel ashamed of their natural desires or appearance, particularly when their experiences do not align with media-driven fantasies.

3. Past Trauma

Experiences of abuse, assault, or other negative touch can have profound and lasting effects on an individual's relationship with their body and intimacy. Trauma often creates associations between touch and harm, making it difficult to engage in safe, consensual experiences like sensual massage without feelings of shame or discomfort.

The Body's Response to Trauma

Trauma is stored in the body, often manifesting as hypervigilance, numbness, or pain. Survivors may experience:

- **Hyperarousal:** Heightened sensitivity to touch, leading to feelings of fear or panic.

- **Emotional numbing:** Difficulty connecting with sensations or emotions during physical touch.

- **Flashbacks:** Physical touch may trigger memories of past abuse, evoking shame or fear.

The Role of Shame in Trauma

Shame is a common response to trauma, as survivors often internalize blame or believe they are damaged or unworthy. This shame can make it challenging to seek healing through practices like sensual massage, which require vulnerability and trust.

4. Fear of Vulnerability

Sensual massage often requires individuals to be vulnerable—both physically and emotionally. This vulnerability can unearth insecurities, fears, and deeply buried shame.

Physical Vulnerability

The act of undressing or allowing another person to touch one's body can evoke feelings of exposure or embarrassment. Individuals may fear being judged for their appearance, weight, scars, or other perceived imperfections.

Emotional Vulnerability

Sensual massage goes beyond physical touch; it often brings emotions to the surface. For some, the prospect of confronting buried feelings—such as grief, anger, or longing—can be overwhelming. This fear of emotional exposure may lead to avoidance or resistance, reinforcing shame.

Manifestations of Shame in the Human Experience

Shame does not exist in isolation; it affects multiple dimensions of an individual's life, including their mental health, relationships, and sense of self-worth.

1. Psychological Effects

Shame is closely linked to mental health conditions such as:

- **Depression:** Persistent feelings of unworthiness or inadequacy can lead to hopelessness and despair.

- **Anxiety:** Fear of judgment or rejection often accompanies shame, contributing to social withdrawal.

- **Low self-esteem:** Shame erodes confidence, making it difficult to assert boundaries or pursue personal goals.

2. Relational Effects

Shame often interferes with the ability to form healthy, intimate relationships. It can lead to:

- **Avoidance:** Individuals may withdraw from touch or intimacy to protect themselves from perceived judgment.

- **Conflict:** Shame can manifest as defensiveness or anger in relationships, creating distance.

- **Insecurity:** A fear of being "not enough" may result in clinginess or co-dependency.

3. Physical Effects

Chronic shame can have physiological consequences, including:

- **Tension:** Holding shame in the body can lead to tightness in the shoulders, jaw, or chest.

- **Fatigue:** The emotional toll of shame can leave individuals feeling drained.

- **Health issues:** Prolonged stress associated with shame can contribute to conditions such as high blood pressure or immune dysfunction.

Healing Shame Through Sensuality

Despite its profound impact, shame is not insurmountable. Practices like sensual massage offer a pathway to healing by fostering self-acceptance, connection, and trust.

1. Reclaiming the Body

Sensual massage encourages individuals to reconnect with their bodies in a nurturing and non-judgmental way. It promotes:

- **Awareness:** Paying attention to physical sensations helps individuals move from a place of disconnection to one of presence.

- **Acceptance:** By experiencing touch as safe and affirming, individuals can begin to view their bodies as worthy of care and appreciation.

2. Establishing Safe Boundaries

Consent and communication are central to sensual massage. These practices teach individuals to:

- **Set boundaries:** Clearly articulating needs and limits helps foster a sense of safety.

- **Respect others:** Learning to navigate boundaries with a partner builds trust and mutual understanding.

3. Releasing Stored Emotions

Sensual touch can release emotions that have been stored in the body. By creating a safe space for expression, individuals can process and let go of shame, grief, or anger.

4. Embracing Vulnerability

Vulnerability is an antidote to shame. Sensual massage allows individuals to practice vulnerability in a controlled and supportive environment, gradually replacing fear with confidence and trust.

Conclusion

Shame is a universal emotion that profoundly influences the human experience, particularly in matters of sensuality, intimacy, and touch. Its origins are multifaceted, rooted in cultural conditioning, societal expectations, past trauma, and fears of vulnerability. While shame can be deeply ingrained, it is not insurmountable.

By addressing the sources of shame and embracing practices like sensual massage, individuals can begin to heal their relationship with their bodies, emotions, and sense of self-worth. Through intentional touch, communication, and mindfulness, sensual massage offers a pathway to reclaiming joy, connection, and authenticity in the face of shame.

Understanding and confronting shame is a transformative journey—one that leads not only to personal liberation but also to deeper, more meaningful relationships with others and oneself.

Shame is a pervasive and deeply rooted emotion that often causes individuals to disconnect from their bodies, emotions, and sense of self-worth. It thrives in secrecy, avoidance, and judgment, creating barriers to intimacy and self-acceptance. Sensual massage offers a unique and powerful way to confront and heal shame through intentional touch, mutual consent, and mindfulness. By encouraging vulnerability and fostering connection, sensual massage allows individuals to reframe their relationship with their body, emotions, and identity.

In this article, we explore how sensual massage challenges and dissolves shame, focusing on its transformative impact in four key areas:

reclaiming the body, establishing safe boundaries, encouraging vulnerability, and healing emotional wounds.

---

1. Reclaiming the Body

One of the most profound effects of shame is the disconnect it creates between individuals and their bodies. Shame often teaches us to view our physical form as flawed, unworthy, or a source of discomfort. Sensual massage offers a safe and nurturing way to reclaim the body as a source of pleasure, empowerment, and self-expression.

Awareness: Connecting with the Body

Sensual massage encourages individuals to focus on physical sensations without judgment. This mindful awareness helps bridge the gap between the mind and body, allowing individuals to:

- **Reconnect with sensations:** Paying attention to the warmth, pressure, and rhythm of touch can help individuals feel present and grounded.

- **Interrupt negative thought patterns:** By focusing on sensory experiences, individuals can shift their attention away from critical or shaming self-talk.

For those who have long felt disconnected from their body—whether due to societal pressure, trauma, or personal insecurities—this process can be a revelation.

Acceptance: Celebrating the Body's Potential

Sensual massage creates a non-judgmental space where individuals can experience their body's capacity for relaxation and pleasure. This environment fosters self-acceptance by:

- **Challenging societal standards:** Participants are encouraged to appreciate their body as it is, rather than comparing it to idealized beauty standards.

- **Acknowledging the body's strengths:** Sensual massage highlights the body's ability to feel, heal, and connect, shifting the focus from appearance to function and sensation.

This reframing can be particularly transformative for individuals who have experienced body-related shame. Over time, they may develop a sense of ownership and pride in their physical form.

2. Establishing Safe Boundaries

Consent and communication are cornerstones of sensual massage. For individuals burdened by shame—especially those whose boundaries have been violated in the past—this emphasis on safety and respect can be revolutionary.

The Importance of Clear Communication

Before a sensual massage session begins, practitioners and participants discuss comfort levels, boundaries, and expectations. This open dialogue ensures that:

- **Consent is explicit:** Every aspect of the experience is agreed upon, eliminating ambiguity or coercion.

- **Participants feel empowered:** The ability to set and enforce boundaries reinforces a sense of control and autonomy.

This process not only fosters trust but also demonstrates that intimacy can exist without pressure or discomfort.

The Healing Power of Respect

Many individuals who struggle with shame have experienced boundary violations in the past, whether through trauma, societal pressure, or unhealthy relationships. Sensual massage provides a contrasting experience—one where:

- **Touch is respectful and intentional:** Every action is guided by the recipient's comfort and preferences.

- **Boundaries are celebrated:** The act of setting limits is seen as a sign of self-awareness and strength, rather than a hindrance to connection.

This respectful dynamic can help individuals rebuild their capacity for trust and intimacy.

---

3. Encouraging Vulnerability

Shame thrives in secrecy and avoidance, feeding off the fear of judgment and rejection. Sensual massage challenges this cycle by creating a space where vulnerability is welcomed and supported.

Confronting Discomfort

For many individuals, the act of receiving or giving sensual touch can feel intimidating. It requires a level of openness—both physical and emotional—that shame often suppresses. Sensual massage helps participants confront this discomfort by:

- **Normalizing vulnerability:** The practice frames openness as a strength rather than a weakness.

- **Providing reassurance:** A supportive environment helps individuals feel safe enough to face their fears.

Over time, this exposure can reduce the power of shame, replacing it with confidence and self-assurance.

Fostering Connection

Vulnerability is not only about confronting fear; it's also about creating meaningful connections. Sensual massage encourages participants to:

- **Express their needs:** Open communication fosters a sense of mutual understanding and empathy.

- **Receive care without guilt:** Allowing oneself to be cared for without self-criticism is a key step toward overcoming shame.

This process helps individuals see vulnerability as a pathway to deeper relationships, rather than a risk to be avoided.

---

4. Healing Emotional Wounds

Emotions are often stored in the body, particularly when they are tied to trauma, shame, or unresolved conflicts. Sensual massage offers a unique way to access and release these buried feelings, providing an opportunity for healing and growth.

Releasing Stored Tension

The body often holds onto emotional pain in the form of physical tension. Sensual massage can help release this tension by:

- **Activating the parasympathetic nervous system:** Gentle, rhythmic touch calms the body, making it easier to let go of stress and fear.

- **Loosening muscle tightness:** By working through areas of physical restriction, the practice can free trapped emotions.

This release often leads to a sense of lightness, clarity, and emotional balance.

Processing Buried Feelings

As the body relaxes, emotions that have been suppressed may come to the surface. Sensual massage creates a safe environment for processing these feelings, allowing individuals to:

- **Acknowledge their emotions:** Naming and recognizing feelings is the first step toward healing.

- **Express their experiences:** Whether through tears, laughter, or verbal sharing, participants can release emotions in a supportive setting.

This emotional catharsis can be transformative, helping individuals feel more connected to themselves and others.

Practical Steps for Using Sensual Massage to Address Shame

For those interested in exploring sensual massage as a tool for healing shame, the following steps can help ensure a positive and empowering experience:

1. Start with Self-Massage

Self-massage is an excellent way to build comfort with touch and explore sensations in a private, judgment-free space. Techniques include:

- Using oils to massage areas like the arms, legs, and feet.

- Practicing mindfulness by focusing on the sensations of touch.

- Repeating affirmations to foster self-acceptance (e.g., "My body is worthy of care and love").

2. Choose a Trustworthy Partner or Practitioner

If working with a partner or professional, it's essential to establish trust and rapport. Look for someone who:

- Respects your boundaries and values consent.

- Creates a safe and supportive environment.

- Communicates openly about expectations and goals.

3. Create a Relaxing Environment

The setting plays a crucial role in sensual massage. Elements like soft lighting, calming music, and scented oils can enhance the experience and promote relaxation.

4. Practice Open Communication

Whether with a partner or practitioner, clear communication is key. Discuss:

- Your comfort levels and boundaries.

- Any areas of physical or emotional sensitivity.

- Your goals for the experience (e.g., relaxation, emotional release, intimacy).

Real-Life Transformations Through Sensual Massage

The transformative power of sensual massage is evident in the stories of individuals who have used the practice to confront and heal shame:

Anna's Journey to Self-Acceptance

Anna, a survivor of childhood trauma, struggled with feelings of unworthiness and body shame. Through guided sensual massage, she learned to view her body as a source of strength and resilience. Over time, the practice helped her rebuild trust in herself and embrace her vulnerability as a sign of courage.

Mark and Lisa's Rediscovery of Intimacy

Mark and Lisa, a married couple, had grown distant after years of stress and unspoken resentment. Sensual massage allowed them to reconnect by fostering open communication and mutual care. The practice helped them replace shame and defensiveness with trust and intimacy.

Raj's Liberation from Body Image Shame

Raj, who had long felt ashamed of his weight and appearance, began exploring self-massage as a way to confront his insecurities. The practice helped him develop a newfound appreciation for his body's capabilities, transforming his relationship with himself and others.

Conclusion

Sensual massage is a powerful tool for challenging and healing shame. By fostering awareness, acceptance, vulnerability, and connection, it allows individuals to confront their fears, embrace their bodies, and process buried emotions in a supportive environment. Through this practice, shame can be replaced with empowerment, self-love, and a deeper sense of belonging.

As more people explore the healing potential of sensual massage, its transformative effects can extend beyond individuals, contributing to a broader cultural shift toward acceptance, openness, and compassion. Whether practiced alone, with a partner, or under professional guidance, sensual massage offers a pathway to liberation from the confines of shame and a celebration of the body's innate capacity for pleasure and connection.

Practical Tips for Overcoming Shame Through Sensual Massage

Shame is a deeply rooted emotion that can create barriers to self-acceptance, intimacy, and emotional well-being. Sensual massage offers a pathway to healing by fostering a positive relationship with the body and emotions. Through intentional touch, mindfulness, and connection, sensual massage creates a safe space to confront and release shame. For those seeking to embrace this practice, starting with practical steps can make the journey manageable and transformative.

This article explores four key strategies to overcome shame through sensual massage: starting with self-massage, focusing on communication, creating a safe space, and seeking professional guidance. These practical tips offer a roadmap for building self-confidence, fostering intimacy, and cultivating a deeper sense of self-acceptance.

---

1. Start with Self-Massage

For individuals who feel hesitant or ashamed, self-massage is an excellent starting point. It provides a private, judgment-free environment where one can explore their body and emotions without external pressure or expectations.

The Benefits of Self-Massage

- **Privacy:** Self-massage allows individuals to work through their feelings of shame or discomfort at their own pace.

- **Empowerment:** Taking control of one's own healing process fosters a sense of agency and confidence.

- **Body Awareness:** Self-massage helps individuals reconnect with their physical sensations, promoting mindfulness and self-acceptance.

Creating the Right Atmosphere

Setting the stage for self-massage is crucial to creating an environment of relaxation and self-love. Consider the following elements:

- **Lighting:** Dim lighting or candlelight can create a soothing ambiance.

- **Aromatherapy:** Essential oils like lavender, chamomile, or sandalwood can enhance relaxation and sensory awareness.

- **Music:** Calming music or nature sounds can help quiet the mind and promote mindfulness.

- **Comfortable Space:** Use soft blankets, cushions, or a massage table to create a supportive and cozy setting.

Techniques for Self-Massage

- **Warm-Up with Oils:** Warm a small amount of oil (e.g., coconut or jojoba oil) in your hands and gently apply it to your skin.

- **Focus on Tension Areas:** Use light to medium pressure to massage areas like the shoulders, neck, arms, and legs.

- **Incorporate Mindfulness:** Pay attention to the sensations of touch, breathing deeply to stay present in the moment.

- **Use Tools if Needed:** Massage balls or rollers can help reach areas like the back or feet.

Affirmations to Encourage Self-Love

During self-massage, repeating affirmations can help counteract negative self-talk. Examples include:

- "My body is worthy of care and love."

- "I release shame and embrace self-acceptance."

- "I honour my body's strength and resilience."

---

2. Focus on Communication

For those exploring sensual massage with a partner, communication is the cornerstone of a positive and healing experience. Open and honest dialogue helps establish trust, set boundaries, and reduce feelings of shame or fear.

The Role of Communication in Overcoming Shame

Shame often thrives in secrecy and avoidance. By openly discussing desires, fears, and boundaries, individuals can:

- **Normalize Vulnerability:** Sharing openly helps reduce the stigma associated with shame.

- **Build Trust:** Clear communication fosters mutual understanding and respect between partners.

- **Ensure Comfort:** Discussing preferences ensures that both partners feel safe and supported.

Topics to Discuss Before Starting

- **Boundaries:** Talk about areas of the body that are off-limits or particularly sensitive.

- **Intentions:** Discuss the goals of the massage (e.g., relaxation, intimacy, emotional release).

- **Comfort Levels:** Share any concerns or insecurities to create a sense of safety.

Tips for Effective Communication

1. **Choose the Right Time:** Have the conversation in a calm and private setting where both partners can focus on the discussion.

2. **Use "I" Statements:** Frame your feelings and needs in a way that avoids blaming or pressuring the other person (e.g., "I feel

nervous about this" rather than "You make me uncomfortable").

3. **Be Patient:** Allow time for each partner to express their thoughts and feelings without rushing or interrupting.

4. **Revisit the Conversation:** Check in periodically during and after the massage to ensure ongoing comfort and satisfaction.

---

3. Create a Safe Space

The environment in which sensual massage takes place significantly impacts the emotional and physical experience. A safe and comfortable setting can help individuals feel more at ease, reducing the power of shame and encouraging relaxation.

The Importance of Safety and Comfort

- **Promotes Relaxation:** A calm environment allows the body and mind to release tension.

- **Reduces Fear of Judgment:** A private, inviting space helps individuals feel secure in their vulnerability.

- **Encourages Presence:** The right atmosphere supports mindfulness and immersion in the experience.

Elements of a Safe Space

1. **Privacy:** Choose a location where interruptions are unlikely, such as a quiet room with a closed door.

2. **Temperature:** Ensure the room is warm enough for comfort, as nudity or minimal clothing may be involved.

3. **Lighting:** Soft, dim lighting creates a calming ambiance and reduces self-consciousness.

4. **Aromatherapy:** Use a diffuser with essential oils to create a soothing and pleasant scent.

5. **Sound:** Play gentle music or nature sounds to mask outside noise and enhance relaxation.

Incorporating Rituals for Mindfulness

Rituals can help set the tone for a sensual massage, signalling to the mind and body that it's time to relax and let go of shame. Examples include:

- **Meditative Breathing:** Begin with a few minutes of deep breathing to centre yourself.

- **Intentions:** Set a positive intention for the session, such as "I will embrace my body with love and kindness."

- **Grounding Practices:** Use grounding techniques like visualizing roots growing from your feet to anchor yourself in the present moment.

---

4. Seek Professional Guidance

For individuals dealing with significant shame or trauma, seeking the support of a certified sensual massage therapist or somatic healer can be transformative. These professionals are trained to navigate the emotional complexities that may arise during the practice, providing a safe and supportive environment for healing.

The Benefits of Professional Guidance

- **Expertise:** Professionals have the knowledge and experience to address physical and emotional needs effectively.

- **Objectivity:** Working with a professional removes the pressure of managing emotions or expectations with a partner.

- **Supportive Environment:** Therapists create a structured, judgment-free space where clients can explore their feelings safely.

Choosing the Right Professional

When seeking a sensual massage therapist or somatic healer, consider the following factors:

1. **Certifications and Training:** Look for practitioners with credentials in massage therapy, somatic healing, or trauma-informed care.

2. **Reputation:** Read reviews or ask for recommendations to ensure the practitioner is reputable and ethical.

3. **Comfort Level:** Choose someone with whom you feel comfortable and safe. Many therapists offer consultations to discuss goals and address concerns before the session.

What to Expect in a Professional Session

- **Intake Discussion:** The session typically begins with a conversation about your needs, boundaries, and expectations.

- **Customized Approach:** The therapist tailors the massage to your comfort level, incorporating techniques that align with your goals.

- **Ongoing Communication:** The therapist checks in regularly during the session to ensure your comfort and consent.

Working Through Emotional Releases

It's not uncommon for individuals to experience emotional releases during or after a sensual massage session, such as crying, laughter, or feelings of relief. A trained professional can help you navigate these emotions, offering guidance and support as you process them.

Integrating Sensual Massage into Daily Life

Overcoming shame is a journey, not a one-time event. By integrating sensual massage into your routine, you can continue to build self-confidence, deepen intimacy, and foster emotional resilience.

Incorporate Self-Care Practices

- Use self-massage as part of your daily routine to maintain a connection with your body.

- Combine massage with other self-care rituals, such as yoga, journaling, or meditation.

Strengthen Relationships Through Touch

- Make sensual massage a regular practice with your partner to nurture intimacy and trust.

- Use the principles of communication and consent in all aspects of your relationship.

Celebrate Progress

- Acknowledge and celebrate small victories, such as feeling more comfortable with touch or expressing your needs.

- Reflect on how far you've come in your journey to overcome shame, using these milestones as motivation to continue.

Conclusion

Sensual massage is a powerful tool for confronting and overcoming shame. By starting with self-massage, fostering open communication, creating a safe space, and seeking professional guidance, individuals can embark on a transformative journey toward self-acceptance and emotional healing. Each step offers an opportunity to reconnect with the body, release negative emotions, and embrace vulnerability with courage and grace.

The process of overcoming shame through sensual massage is deeply personal, but its benefits extend far beyond the individual. By fostering self-love and emotional resilience, this practice has the potential to transform relationships, build trust, and promote a more compassionate understanding of the human experience. Whether practiced alone, with a partner, or under professional guidance, sensual massage offers a pathway to liberation and a celebration of the body's innate wisdom and beauty.

Addressing Misconceptions and Reducing Stigma

Sensual massage is often misunderstood and stigmatized due to its association with sexuality. However, educating others about its therapeutic and healing aspects can shift perceptions. Efforts to normalize sensual touch include:

- **Advocacy:** Highlighting stories of healing and transformation to dispel myths.

- **Education:** Offering workshops and resources about the benefits and ethics of sensual massage.

- **Inclusivity:** Emphasizing that sensual massage is for everyone, regardless of gender, age, or relationship status.

Addressing Misconceptions and Reducing Stigma: Sensual Massage in Focus

Sensual massage is a multifaceted practice with profound therapeutic and emotional benefits. Yet, despite its potential to heal and transform, it remains shrouded in misunderstanding and stigma, largely due to its association with sexuality. These misconceptions often prevent individuals from exploring its benefits or openly discussing their experiences with it.

By reframing sensual massage as a tool for healing, connection, and self-awareness, society can begin to normalize this practice. Advocacy, education, and inclusivity are key strategies in reducing stigma and fostering greater understanding of sensual massage. This article explores the origins of misconceptions, the impact of stigma, and actionable steps to change societal attitudes.

Understanding Misconceptions Surrounding Sensual Massage

The stigma surrounding sensual massage is deeply rooted in cultural, societal, and historical factors. To address these misconceptions, it's essential to understand their origins and manifestations.

1. The Association with Sexuality

Sensual massage is often conflated with sexual activity due to its focus on touch, intimacy, and relaxation. While sensual massage can incorporate elements of pleasure, its purpose is not inherently sexual. This misunderstanding arises from:

- **Cultural taboos:** Many societies view touch, particularly intimate or erogenous touch, as inherently sexual and therefore taboo.

- **Media portrayals:** Popular culture often sensationalizes or misrepresents sensual massage, perpetuating the idea that it is exclusively a form of sexual service.

- **Lack of education:** The absence of clear distinctions between sensual massage, therapeutic massage, and sexual activity contributes to widespread confusion.

2. Fear of Vulnerability

Sensual massage often requires individuals to be physically and emotionally open, which can feel intimidating. This vulnerability is sometimes misinterpreted as a sign of impropriety or weakness, further perpetuating stigma.

3. Gender Stereotypes

Cultural norms around gender and touch also fuel misconceptions. For example:

- Men may be stigmatized for seeking sensual massage due to stereotypes that associate male vulnerability with weakness.

- Women may face judgment for embracing sensual touch, as societal norms often shame female expressions of sensuality.

The Impact of Stigma on Individuals and Society

The stigma surrounding sensual massage has far-reaching consequences, both for individuals and the broader community.

1. Barriers to Healing and Connection

Many individuals who could benefit from sensual massage avoid it due to fear of judgment or misunderstanding. This hesitation can prevent them from:

- Releasing emotional tension and trauma.

- Building intimacy with themselves or their partners.

- Exploring non-sexual forms of pleasure and relaxation.

2. Isolation and Shame

The lack of open dialogue about sensual massage fosters isolation and shame, making it difficult for individuals to discuss their experiences or seek guidance.

3. Limited Access to Education and Resources

The stigma also hinders the development and accessibility of educational materials, workshops, and professional training related to sensual massage.

Shifting Perceptions: Advocacy, Education, and Inclusivity

To address misconceptions and reduce stigma, society must adopt proactive strategies that highlight the therapeutic and healing aspects of sensual massage. Advocacy, education, and inclusivity play pivotal roles in this effort.

---

1. Advocacy: Highlighting Stories of Healing and Transformation

Advocacy is a powerful tool for changing perceptions and normalizing sensual massage. Sharing personal stories and testimonials can humanize the practice and dispel myths.

The Power of Personal Stories

- **Humanizing the experience:** Stories of individuals who have healed emotional wounds, improved their relationships, or deepened their self-awareness through sensual massage can challenge stereotypes and misconceptions.

- **Building empathy:** Hearing about others' transformative experiences fosters understanding and reduces judgment.

Examples of Advocacy Efforts

- **Social media campaigns:** Platforms like Instagram, YouTube, and TikTok can be used to share testimonials and educational content.

- **Documentaries and articles:** Highlighting real-life stories in mainstream media can reach a wider audience and normalize the practice.

- **Community events:** Hosting events where individuals can share their experiences and learn from others creates a supportive environment for advocacy.

---

2. Education: Offering Workshops and Resources

Education is essential for dispelling myths and providing accurate information about the benefits, ethics, and practice of sensual massage.

Developing Educational Programs

Workshops, online courses, and in-person events can teach participants about:

- **The history and philosophy of sensual massage:** Understanding its roots in ancient healing practices can help contextualize its purpose.

- **Techniques and approaches:** Demonstrating how sensual massage differs from other forms of massage or touch.

- **The importance of consent and boundaries:** Emphasizing mutual respect and communication in every interaction.

Creating Accessible Resources

Accessible materials, such as books, blogs, and videos, can help demystify sensual massage for a wider audience. Topics might include:

- The physical and emotional benefits of sensual massage.

- Tips for incorporating sensual massage into daily life.

- Addressing common concerns or misconceptions.

Training for Professionals

Providing specialized training for massage therapists and wellness practitioners can ensure they are equipped to navigate the complexities of sensual massage with professionalism and empathy.

---

3. Inclusivity: Emphasizing Universality

One of the most effective ways to reduce stigma is to highlight that sensual massage is for everyone, regardless of gender, age, or relationship status.

Breaking Down Stereotypes

- **For all genders:** Emphasizing that sensual massage is not limited to women or couples can encourage more men and nonbinary individuals to explore its benefits.

- **For all ages:** Sensual massage can benefit individuals at every stage of life, from young adults seeking self-discovery to seniors looking for relaxation and connection.

- **For all relationship statuses:** Sensual massage is not just for couples; it can be practiced solo or with friends in a non-romantic context.

Celebrating Diversity

Representing a diverse range of individuals in educational materials and advocacy efforts can help normalize sensual massage and make it more accessible. This might include:

- Showcasing different body types, ethnicities, and age groups.

- Highlighting the experiences of LGBTQ+ individuals.

- Featuring stories from individuals with disabilities or chronic illnesses who have benefited from sensual massage.

Practical Steps for Reducing Stigma

To complement broader advocacy and educational efforts, individuals can take practical steps to challenge misconceptions and promote understanding in their personal lives and communities.

1. Open Conversations

Talking openly about sensual massage with friends, family, or colleagues can help normalize the topic and reduce fear or judgment.

Tips for Starting the Conversation

- Use neutral language: Frame the discussion around the therapeutic and healing aspects of sensual massage.

- Share personal experiences: If comfortable, discuss how sensual massage has benefited you.

- Address misconceptions: Be prepared to clarify common myths and provide accurate information.

2. Lead by Example

By embracing sensual massage in your own life, you can demonstrate its benefits and encourage others to explore it without fear or shame.

Ways to Lead by Example

- Practice self-massage and share your experiences.

- Invite friends or partners to participate in a workshop or group session.

- Support local practitioners or organizations that promote sensual massage.

---

3. Support Advocacy and Education

Getting involved in advocacy and educational initiatives can amplify your impact and contribute to broader societal change.

How to Get Involved

- Volunteer with organizations that promote body positivity and wellness.

- Share educational resources on social media or in community groups.

- Attend events, workshops, or conferences related to sensual massage and its benefits.

Conclusion

Sensual massage has the potential to transform lives by fostering self-acceptance, connection, and emotional healing. However, misconceptions and stigma often prevent individuals from embracing its benefits. By addressing these misconceptions through advocacy, education, and inclusivity, society can create a more open and supportive environment for this practice.

Through personal stories, accessible resources, and a commitment to diversity, sensual massage can be reframed as a universal and therapeutic practice. As more people embrace its potential, the stigma surrounding sensual massage will gradually diminish, paving the way for a culture that celebrates the healing power of touch.

Re-evaluation and Acceptance: Embracing Sensual Massage Without Shame

Sensual massage is an intimate and transformative experience that has the potential to foster self-awareness, relaxation, and deeper connections. However, for many, it is accompanied by shame—an emotion that can hinder full acceptance and enjoyment of the practice. Reevaluating our perception of sensual massage and cultivating acceptance is a journey that involves examining our internal beliefs, societal influences, and personal boundaries. By reflecting deeply on the sources of our shame, we can move toward a healthier relationship with our bodies, desires, and emotions.

This article explores the steps involved in reevaluating and accepting sensual massage as a practice free from shame. It offers insights into identifying the root causes of shame, reframing sensuality in a positive light, and embracing the experience with authenticity and self-respect.

Understanding the Role of Shame

What Is Shame?

Shame is a deeply ingrained emotion that arises from the belief that we have violated social norms or personal values. Unlike guilt, which focuses on actions, shame targets the self, creating feelings of inadequacy or unworthiness. In the context of sensual massage, shame often stems from societal taboos, personal insecurities, or fear of vulnerability.

Why Does Shame Surround Sensual Massage?

Sensual massage involves touch, intimacy, and the potential for pleasure—elements that are often misunderstood or stigmatized. Common sources of shame include:

- **Cultural conditioning:** Many cultures associate sensuality with immorality or frivolity, creating a fear of judgment.

- **Religious teachings:** Some religious doctrines emphasize modesty and restraint, fostering guilt around physical pleasure.

- **Media influence:** Unrealistic beauty standards and hypersexualized portrayals of touch can distort perceptions of sensuality.

- **Personal insecurities:** Negative self-image or past trauma can make individuals feel uncomfortable with touch or intimacy.

Recognizing these influences is the first step in reevaluating our perspective and working toward acceptance.

Step 1: Deep Reflection on the Causes of Shame

Reevaluating our perception of sensual massage requires a willingness to explore the root causes of our shame. This process involves self-awareness, honesty, and a commitment to growth.

Identifying Internalized Beliefs

Ask yourself the following questions to uncover the beliefs that may be fuelling your shame:

- **What messages did I receive about sensuality growing up?** Reflect on cultural, familial, or religious teachings that shaped your views on touch and intimacy.

- **How do I feel about my body?** Consider whether insecurities or societal standards influence your comfort with sensual experiences.

- **What fears or judgments arise during a sensual massage?** Identify specific thoughts or emotions that trigger discomfort or shame.

By bringing these beliefs to light, you can begin to challenge and reframe them.

Exploring the Role of Past Experiences

Shame often has its roots in past experiences, particularly those involving trauma, rejection, or negative touch. Reflect on:

- **Memories of shame:** Recall instances when you felt judged or unworthy in the context of touch or intimacy.

- **Unresolved emotions:** Consider whether unresolved pain or fear is influencing your current perspective.

Seeking professional support, such as therapy, can be helpful in processing these experiences and moving forward.

Step 2: Reframing Sensuality in a Positive Light

To overcome shame, it's essential to shift your perception of sensuality from something taboo or shameful to something natural and empowering. This involves challenging societal narratives and embracing a more holistic understanding of sensual massage.

Recognizing the Therapeutic Benefits of Sensual Massage

Sensual massage is not solely about pleasure—it's a practice that promotes physical, emotional, and psychological well-being. Its benefits include:

- **Relaxation:** Releasing tension and reducing stress through intentional touch.

- **Emotional healing:** Providing a safe space to process and release stored emotions.

- **Self-awareness:** Enhancing mindfulness and connection to the body.

By focusing on these therapeutic aspects, you can reframe sensual massage as a legitimate and valuable practice.

Celebrating the Body's Capacity for Pleasure

Pleasure is a natural and essential part of the human experience. Sensual massage provides an opportunity to:

- **Appreciate your body:** Focus on what your body can do and feel, rather than how it looks or measures up to societal standards.

- **Reconnect with sensation:** Experience touch as a source of comfort, connection, and joy.

- **Normalize pleasure:** Acknowledge that enjoying sensuality is not shameful but a healthy expression of self-care and intimacy.

This reframing allows you to approach sensual massage with a sense of curiosity and acceptance.

Step 3: Embracing Boundaries and Autonomy

Acceptance of sensual massage does not mean disregarding your boundaries or needs. In fact, setting and respecting boundaries is crucial for creating a sense of safety and comfort.

Defining Your Comfort Levels

Before engaging in a sensual massage, take time to define your personal boundaries. Consider:

- **What areas of the body feel safe or off-limits?**

- **What level of nudity are you comfortable with?**

- **What intentions do you have for the experience (e.g., relaxation, healing, intimacy)?**

Clear boundaries help you feel in control and reduce the likelihood of discomfort or shame.

Communicating Boundaries with Others

If receiving a sensual massage from a partner or professional, communicate your boundaries openly. This dialogue fosters trust and ensures that your needs are respected. Key points to discuss include:

- Areas of sensitivity or vulnerability.

- Preferred techniques or approaches.

- Signals for pausing or stopping the session.

Honouring your autonomy in this way reinforces the idea that sensual massage is a consensual and collaborative experience.

Step 4: Practicing Mindfulness During the Experience

Mindfulness is a powerful tool for overcoming shame and fully embracing the experience of sensual massage. By staying present in the moment, you can quiet self-criticism and focus on the sensations and emotions at hand.

Techniques for Staying Present

- **Deep breathing:** Use slow, intentional breaths to ground yourself and release tension.

- **Body scanning:** Focus on different areas of your body, noticing the sensations without judgment.

- **Positive affirmations:** Repeat affirmations such as, "I am worthy of care and respect," or "It's okay to enjoy this moment."

Mindfulness allows you to approach the experience with curiosity and openness, rather than fear or shame.

Embracing Vulnerability

Sensual massage often involves a degree of vulnerability, both physical and emotional. Instead of resisting this vulnerability, try to embrace it as an opportunity for growth and connection. Vulnerability can:

- Strengthen your relationship with yourself by fostering self-acceptance.

- Deepen your connection with a partner by promoting trust and authenticity.

- Open the door to new experiences and insights.

Step 5: Reevaluating Desires and Needs

Accepting sensual massage also involves reevaluating your own desires and needs. This requires confronting societal judgments and embracing your authenticity.

Letting Go of Judgment

Society often imposes rigid norms about what is "appropriate" when it comes to sensuality and touch. To embrace sensual massage without shame:

- Challenge societal expectations that conflict with your personal values.

- Recognize that your desires and preferences are valid and natural.

- Reject the idea that sensuality is inherently shameful or superficial.

Exploring Your Desires with Openness

Sensual massage is an opportunity to discover what feels pleasurable and meaningful to you. Take time to explore:

- What types of touch or techniques resonate with you.

- How sensual massage aligns with your goals for relaxation, connection, or healing.

- What role intimacy and pleasure play in your overall well-being.

This exploration can lead to greater self-awareness and fulfilment.

Step 6: Fostering a Culture of Acceptance

Individual acceptance of sensual massage is part of a larger cultural shift toward normalizing touch, intimacy, and pleasure. By promoting open dialogue and inclusivity, we can reduce the stigma surrounding sensual massage and create a more supportive environment.

Educating Yourself and Others

Learn about the therapeutic and emotional benefits of sensual massage and share this knowledge with others. Advocacy and education can help challenge misconceptions and promote understanding.

Celebrating Diversity

Sensual massage is for everyone, regardless of age, gender, or relationship status. By embracing diverse perspectives and experiences, we can foster a culture of inclusivity and acceptance.

Encouraging Open Dialogue

Discussing sensual massage openly—whether with friends, partners, or communities—can help normalize the practice and reduce feelings of shame. Sharing personal experiences and insights can also inspire others to explore sensuality in a positive way.

Conclusion: A Path to Self-Acceptance and Fulfilment

Reevaluating and accepting sensual massage are a journey that involves deep reflection, open-mindedness, and self-compassion. By confronting the sources of shame, reframing sensuality as a natural and empowering aspect of life, and embracing your boundaries and needs, you can approach sensual massage with greater confidence and authenticity.

This process is not only a path to greater self-acceptance but also an opportunity to explore intimacy and pleasure in a freer and more fulfilling way. By normalizing sensual massage and fostering a culture of acceptance, we can move closer to a world where touch and connection are celebrated as essential elements of the human experience.

Adam and Eve: Innocence, Shame, and Sensuality

The story of Adam and Eve offers a profound exploration of innocence, shame, and sensuality. It illustrates how the transition from one state to another reshaped their understanding of themselves and their bodies.

Adam and Eve lived in pure innocence before eating the fruit from the Tree of Knowledge. They were naked yet felt no shame, as their perception of the world and themselves was untainted by self-consciousness or judgment. Their bodies were expressions of their divine creation, seen as natural and good, without any notion of imperfection or inadequacy. In this state, they embodied a harmonious relationship with themselves, each other, and their surroundings—a unity of being that transcended the need for self-awareness.

After partaking in the fruit, their innocence was replaced by a sudden awareness of their nakedness. This newfound knowledge introduced shame, marking a fundamental shift in how they perceived their bodies and their relationship with each other. No longer simply accepting their physicality as natural, they became self-conscious, covering themselves with fig leaves and retreating from the openness they once shared. This moment symbolizes the birth of self-judgment and the loss of untainted intimacy.

From a sensual perspective, the story highlights a distinction between innocence and the awakened awareness of one's body and its desires. Before the fruit, one's physicality was a part of one's being, experienced without thought or critique. Afterwards, sensuality became intertwined with knowledge, choice, and the complexity of human emotion—both a source of connection and a potential cause for vulnerability and shame.

The transition in the story invites reflection on how awareness of one's body and sensuality can lead to growth and challenge. It suggests that while innocence is lost, there is an opportunity for reclaiming a more profound connection with oneself and others through understanding and acceptance. In this context, sensuality can be seen not as inherently tied to shame but as a pathway to rediscovering intimacy and appreciation when approached with mindfulness and respect.

Re-evaluation and Acceptance: Embracing Sensual Massage Without Shame

Sensual massage is an intimate and transformative experience that has the potential to foster self-awareness, relaxation, and deeper connections. However, for many, it is accompanied by shame—an emotion that can hinder full acceptance and enjoyment of the practice. Reevaluating our perception of sensual massage and cultivating acceptance is a journey that involves examining our internal beliefs, societal influences, and personal boundaries. By reflecting deeply on the sources of our shame, we can move toward a healthier relationship with our bodies, desires, and emotions.

This article explores the steps involved in reevaluating and accepting sensual massage as a practice free from shame. It offers insights into identifying the root causes of shame, reframing sensuality in a positive light, and embracing the experience with authenticity and self-respect.

Understanding the Role of Shame

What Is Shame?

Shame is a deeply ingrained emotion that arises from the belief that we have violated social norms or personal values. Unlike guilt, which focuses on actions, shame targets the self, creating feelings of inadequacy or unworthiness. In the context of sensual massage, shame often stems from societal taboos, personal insecurities, or fear of vulnerability.

Why Does Shame Surround Sensual Massage?

Sensual massage involves touch, intimacy, and the potential for pleasure—elements that are often misunderstood or stigmatized. Common sources of shame include:

- **Cultural conditioning:** Many cultures associate sensuality with immorality or frivolity, creating a fear of judgment.

- **Religious teachings:** Some religious doctrines emphasize modesty and restraint, fostering guilt around physical pleasure.

- **Media influence:** Unrealistic beauty standards and hypersexualized portrayals of touch can distort perceptions of sensuality.

- **Personal insecurities:** Negative self-image or past trauma can make individuals feel uncomfortable with touch or intimacy.

Recognizing these influences is the first step in reevaluating our perspective and working toward acceptance.

Step 1: Deep Reflection on the Causes of Shame

Reevaluating our perception of sensual massage requires a willingness to explore the root causes of our shame. This process involves self-awareness, honesty, and a commitment to growth.

Identifying Internalized Beliefs

Ask yourself the following questions to uncover the beliefs that may be fuelling your shame:

- **What messages did I receive about sensuality growing up?** Reflect on cultural, familial, or religious teachings that shaped your views on touch and intimacy.

- **How do I feel about my body?** Consider whether insecurities or societal standards influence your comfort with sensual experiences.

- **What fears or judgments arise during a sensual massage?** Identify specific thoughts or emotions that trigger discomfort or shame.

By bringing these beliefs to light, you can begin to challenge and reframe them.

Exploring the Role of Past Experiences

Shame often has its roots in past experiences, particularly those involving trauma, rejection, or negative touch. Reflect on:

- **Memories of shame:** Recall instances when you felt judged or unworthy in the context of touch or intimacy.

- **Unresolved emotions:** Consider whether unresolved pain or fear is influencing your current perspective.

Seeking professional support, such as therapy, can be helpful in processing these experiences and moving forward.

Step 2: Reframing Sensuality in a Positive Light

To overcome shame, it's essential to shift your perception of sensuality from something taboo or shameful to something natural and empowering. This involves challenging societal narratives and embracing a more holistic understanding of sensual massage.

Recognizing the Therapeutic Benefits of Sensual Massage

Sensual massage is not solely about pleasure—it's a practice that promotes physical, emotional, and psychological well-being. Its benefits include:

- **Relaxation:** Releasing tension and reducing stress through intentional touch.

- **Emotional healing:** Providing a safe space to process and release stored emotions.

- **Self-awareness:** Enhancing mindfulness and connection to the body.

By focusing on these therapeutic aspects, you can reframe sensual massage as a legitimate and valuable practice.

Celebrating the Body's Capacity for Pleasure

Pleasure is a natural and essential part of the human experience. Sensual massage provides an opportunity to:

- **Appreciate your body:** Focus on what your body can do and feel, rather than how it looks or measures up to societal standards.

- **Reconnect with sensation:** Experience touch as a source of comfort, connection, and joy.

- **Normalize pleasure:** Acknowledge that enjoying sensuality is not shameful but a healthy expression of self-care and intimacy.

This reframing allows you to approach sensual massage with a sense of curiosity and acceptance.

Step 3: Embracing Boundaries and Autonomy

Acceptance of sensual massage does not mean disregarding your boundaries or needs. In fact, setting and respecting boundaries is crucial for creating a sense of safety and comfort.

Defining Your Comfort Levels

Before engaging in a sensual massage, take time to define your personal boundaries. Consider:

- **What areas of the body feel safe or off-limits?**

- **What level of nudity are you comfortable with?**

- **What intentions do you have for the experience (e.g., relaxation, healing, intimacy)?**

Clear boundaries help you feel in control and reduce the likelihood of discomfort or shame.

Communicating Boundaries with Others

If receiving a sensual massage from a partner or professional, communicate your boundaries openly. This dialogue fosters trust and ensures that your needs are respected. Key points to discuss include:

- Areas of sensitivity or vulnerability.

- Preferred techniques or approaches.

- Signals for pausing or stopping the session.

Honouring your autonomy in this way reinforces the idea that sensual massage is a consensual and collaborative experience.

Step 4: Practicing Mindfulness During the Experience

Mindfulness is a powerful tool for overcoming shame and fully embracing the experience of sensual massage. By staying present in the moment, you can quiet self-criticism and focus on the sensations and emotions at hand.

Techniques for Staying Present

- **Deep breathing:** Use slow, intentional breaths to ground yourself and release tension.

- **Body scanning:** Focus on different areas of your body, noticing the sensations without judgment.

- **Positive affirmations:** Repeat affirmations such as, "I am worthy of care and respect," or "It's okay to enjoy this moment."

Mindfulness allows you to approach the experience with curiosity and openness, rather than fear or shame.

Embracing Vulnerability

Sensual massage often involves a degree of vulnerability, both physical and emotional. Instead of resisting this vulnerability, try to embrace it as an opportunity for growth and connection. Vulnerability can:

- Strengthen your relationship with yourself by fostering self-acceptance.

- Deepen your connection with a partner by promoting trust and authenticity.

- Open the door to new experiences and insights.

Step 5: Reevaluating Desires and Needs

Accepting sensual massage also involves reevaluating your own desires and needs. This requires confronting societal judgments and embracing your authenticity.

Letting Go of Judgment

Society often imposes rigid norms about what is "appropriate" when it comes to sensuality and touch. To embrace sensual massage without shame:

- Challenge societal expectations that conflict with your personal values.

- Recognize that your desires and preferences are valid and natural.

- Reject the idea that sensuality is inherently shameful or superficial.

Exploring Your Desires with Openness

Sensual massage is an opportunity to discover what feels pleasurable and meaningful to you. Take time to explore:

- What types of touch or techniques resonate with you.

- How sensual massage aligns with your goals for relaxation, connection, or healing.

- What role intimacy and pleasure play in your overall well-being.

This exploration can lead to greater self-awareness and fulfilment.

Step 6: Fostering a Culture of Acceptance

Individual acceptance of sensual massage is part of a larger cultural shift toward normalizing touch, intimacy, and pleasure. By promoting open dialogue and inclusivity, we can reduce the stigma surrounding sensual massage and create a more supportive environment.

Educating Yourself and Others

Learn about the therapeutic and emotional benefits of sensual massage and share this knowledge with others. Advocacy and education can help challenge misconceptions and promote understanding.

Celebrating Diversity

Sensual massage is for everyone, regardless of age, gender, or relationship status. By embracing diverse perspectives and experiences, we can foster a culture of inclusivity and acceptance.

Encouraging Open Dialogue

Discussing sensual massage openly—whether with friends, partners, or communities—can help normalize the practice and reduce feelings of shame. Sharing personal experiences and insights can also inspire others to explore sensuality in a positive way.

Conclusion: A Path to Self-Acceptance and Fulfilment

Reevaluating and accepting sensual massage are a journey that involves deep reflection, open-mindedness, and self-compassion. By confronting the sources of shame, reframing sensuality as a natural and empowering aspect of life, and embracing your boundaries and needs, you can approach sensual massage with greater confidence and authenticity.

This process is not only a path to greater self-acceptance but also an opportunity to explore intimacy and pleasure in a freer and more fulfilling way. By normalizing sensual massage and fostering a culture of acceptance, we can move closer to a world where touch and connection are celebrated as essential elements of the human experience.

Adam and Eve: Innocence, Shame, and Sensuality

The story of Adam and Eve offers a profound exploration of innocence, shame, and sensuality. It illustrates how the transition from one state to another reshaped their understanding of themselves and their bodies.

Adam and Eve lived in pure innocence before eating the fruit from the Tree of Knowledge. They were naked yet felt no shame, as their perception of the world and themselves was untainted by self-consciousness or judgment. Their bodies were expressions of their divine creation, seen as natural and good, without any notion of imperfection or inadequacy. In this state, they embodied a harmonious relationship with themselves, each other, and their surroundings—a unity of being that transcended the need for self-awareness.

After partaking in the fruit, their innocence was replaced by a sudden awareness of their nakedness. This newfound knowledge introduced shame, marking a fundamental shift in how they perceived their bodies and their relationship with each other. No longer simply accepting their physicality as natural, they became self-conscious, covering themselves with fig leaves and retreating from the openness they once shared. This moment symbolizes the birth of self-judgment and the loss of untainted intimacy.

From a sensual perspective, the story highlights a distinction between innocence and the awakened awareness of one's body and its desires. Before the fruit, one's physicality was a part of one's being, experienced without thought or critique. Afterwards, sensuality became intertwined with knowledge, choice, and the complexity of human emotion—both a source of connection and a potential cause for vulnerability and shame.

The transition in the story invites reflection on how awareness of one's body and sensuality can lead to growth and challenge. It suggests that while innocence is lost, there is an opportunity for reclaiming a more profound connection with oneself and others through understanding and acceptance. In this context, sensuality can be seen not as inherently tied to shame but as a pathway to rediscovering intimacy and appreciation when approached with mindfulness and respect.

Adam and Eve: Exploring the Transition from Innocence to Awareness about Modern Sensuality

The narrative of Adam and Eve encapsulates a profound shift from a state of innocence to one of self-awareness, shame, and complexity. This transition can be explored through the lens of modern sensuality and its impact on our relationship with ourselves and others.

1. **Innocence and Unity: A Prelapsarian State**

Before consuming the fruit of knowledge, Adam and Eve existed in harmony with themselves, each other, and creation. Their nakedness was a natural state devoid of self-consciousness or judgment. This innocence symbolizes a pure form of existence, where sensuality—if present—was experienced as an intrinsic part of life, unburdened by shame or desire.

In this state, the body was simply an extension of being, not an object of scrutiny or differentiation. It aligns with childlike innocence, where physicality is experienced without preconceived notions of beauty, worth, or societal constructs.

1. **The Awakening: Knowledge, Shame, and Self-Consciousness**

The act of eating the forbidden fruit symbolizes the acquisition of knowledge—a double-edged gift that brings awareness and consequence. For Adam and Eve, this awareness introduced shame, particularly regarding their bodies. They suddenly perceived their nakedness as something to be hidden, reflecting a new vulnerability and self-consciousness.

This moment parallels how sensuality is often experienced in modern society. As individuals become aware of their bodies and desires, they are simultaneously introduced to societal standards, expectations, and potential judgments. Shame becomes a learned response, often overshadowing the natural appreciation of the body and its capacity for connection and pleasure.

1. The Role of Sensuality: Between Shame and Redemption

In the narrative, the transition from innocence to awareness can be seen as a metaphor for the human journey with sensuality. While shame entered the story after the fruit, it is not sensuality itself that is the source of shame but the context in which it is understood and experienced.

Modern interpretations suggest that sensuality—when approached with mindfulness and respect—has the potential to transcend shame and restore a sense of wholeness. By embracing sensuality as a natural part of human experience, individuals can reclaim a positive relationship with their bodies and desires. It involves:

- **Mindfulness:** Developing a deeper awareness of one's physical and emotional responses, much like Adam and Eve's initial unity with themselves before the fall.

- **Acceptance:** Moving beyond societal judgments to appreciate the body as beautiful, capable, and deserving of care.

- **Connection:** Using sensuality to foster intimacy and trust, not only with others but also within oneself.

1. **Rediscovering Eden: The Path to Integration**

While Adam and Eve's story represents a loss of innocence, it also offers a framework for redemption. Modern approaches to sensuality can focus on integrating the knowledge of the body with self-acceptance, moving from shame to celebration. It requires unlearning harmful narratives about the body and embracing its capacity for pleasure, healing, and connection.

In a broader sense, the narrative invites us to reflect on the balance between awareness and innocence. Rather than returning to a state of naivety, we can aim for an enlightened innocence that combines knowledge with compassion and self-love. This way, sensuality becomes a path to healing and empowerment, not a source of shame.

The Alexandra's story

If someone had told me a few years ago that I would experience sensual massage and end up talking openly about it, I would probably have laughed nervously. Not because I didn't understand the concept but because I could never have imagined myself in the position of facing the deep shame I had about my own body and the idea of pleasure. Now, at 35, I can look back and identify the moment when shame marked my life, transforming into an invisible wall that blocked any attempt to feel free.

I grew up in a traditional family, in a small town where discussions about the body or sensuality were almost non-existent. These topics were not only avoided but practically demonized. The only times they were brought up were accompanied by warnings about decency, morality, and "what others will say." I clearly remember my mother telling me to stand up straight, not to wear too short clothes, and always to be "proper." Any act that seemed "too loose" was seen as a reflection of a lack of respect for myself and my family.

As I grew older, these messages deepened. At school, sex education classes—if I can call them that—were more like fear lessons. They only talked about the consequences of "mistakes"—unwanted pregnancies, sexually transmitted diseases, and the shame that would follow if someone found out. Pleasure, the joy of understanding your body, or intimacy was utterly absent from the conversation. Gradually, I internalized the idea that any exploration of my body or any discussion of desires was inappropriate.

As I reached adolescence, my body became a constant source of discomfort. The changes I was going through—which should have been natural and accepted—made me feel exposed. I was ashamed of every minor imperfection: pimples, the shape of my breasts, the way my legs looked. It felt like everyone was observing and judging every detail, even though, it was just the critical voice in my head.

I remember how I avoided looking in the mirror too much. If I had to get dressed in the shared gym locker room, I would do my best to change as quickly as possible. I was constantly concerned about how others saw me, but I never had a moment to ask myself: "How do I see myself?"

The shame became even more evident as I grew older and entered my first romantic relationship. I remember the first time a boy complimented me—I felt my cheeks flush and wondered if he was sincere or just making fun of me. Compliments, instead of making me feel good, made me feel uncomfortable.

As my relationships became more intimate, things got complicated. I was afraid to express what I wanted, to talk about what made me feel good, or to say what made me feel uncomfortable. I was constantly scared that my desires would be considered "too weird" or "inappropriate." This fear caused me to avoid many meaningful conversations, and my silence created distance in relationships.

"I often shut myself away," I remember now. I told myself it was better to remain silent than risk being judged. But this silence only fuelled the feeling that something was wrong with me.

Shame became a significant barrier in my life. It wasn't just about how I saw myself or related to others but about my relationship with my body. I was ashamed to wear clothes that showed off my body shape, to go to the beach, or to take my shirt off in front of someone. Even in the privacy of my own home, I avoided looking in the mirror.

This shame was like an invisible wall that kept me away from myself. Not only could I not enjoy intimate experiences, but I couldn't even accept them as natural. I often told myself that I didn't deserve to feel good or explore myself, and this thinking deeply affected my self-confidence.

Another factor that intensified my shame was the influence of the media. In magazines, on social media, and in movies, women were presented as idealized, and sensuality always seemed linked to perfection. Any imperfection seemed unacceptable.

I would look at those images and constantly compare myself. I told myself that if I didn't look like those women, then I didn't deserve to enjoy my body. These unrealistic standards made me feel like I was "defective"—never good enough, never attractive enough.

The moment I realized how much shame affected me was simple but powerful. I was in a conversation with my friend Ioana, who was talking so naturally about the body and pleasure. She was telling me about how she had begun to explore sensual massage as a way to connect with herself. At first, I felt a wave of discomfort. It seemed to me that she was talking about something taboo, something that I didn't should be discussed. But at the same time, I also felt a twinge of curiosity. I listened to her story and asked myself, "Why am I feeling so uncomfortable? What would stop me from trying something similar?"

This question got me thinking and became the first step towards awareness. I realized that shame was not a "given" but something I had learned over time—something that could be unlearned.

After that conversation, I decided I didn't want to live in that constant discomfort. I started reading about shame, how it affects people, and how it can be overcome. I started writing in a journal, analysing my thoughts, and asking myself questions.

One of the questions that changed my perspective was, "If no one judged me, what would I do differently?" The answer was clear: I would try to get to know myself better, accept my body, and explore my desires without fear.

This process took work. There were times when old thoughts would come back—thoughts that told me I was putting myself out there too much and that I was at risk of being judged. But gradually, I learned to recognize these thoughts as mental barriers, not absolute truths.

Looking back, I realize that encountering shame was a pivotal moment. Recognizing it wasn't easy, but it was the first step toward freedom. I learned that shame lives in silence, and I can reduce its power by talking about it.

Today, I am grateful for that moment of awareness. It was the beginning of a transformative journey that brought me closer to who I truly am—a person who deserves to feel accessible, connected, and completely authentic.

My transformation began in a completely unexpected way during a seemingly ordinary conversation with my friend Ioana. Ioana was different. She was open to topics that I avoided or didn't even dare to think about too much. She spoke with a natural confidence about the body, about intimacy, and about what seemed to me to be forbidden territory: pleasure and connection with one's own body.

One day, while we were sitting over coffee, Ioana started telling me about a recent experience that, she said, changed her life. "I tried sensual massage," she told me without the slightest trace of embarrassment. For a few seconds, I was speechless. Sensual massage? My mind immediately ran to the preconceived ideas I had about the subject. Many thoughts were running through my head: How can she talk about this so casually? What kind of massage could this be? Is it safe?

I tried to hide my reaction, but Ioana was paying attention. "I know what you're thinking," she said with a smile. "I had the same questions at first. But sensual massage is not what you probably imagine. It's more about healing, about connecting with yourself, than anything else."

I must admit that I was sceptical. Sensual massage sounded like something entirely outside my comfort zone. To me, it was a taboo subject, shrouded in a heavy dose of shame. I grew up believing that such things were either inappropriate or risky. "It's not something I could ever do," I told Ioana, almost defensively. "I'm not the kind of person who feels comfortable with something like that."

Ioana looked at me calmly. "I didn't think that about myself either," she replied. "But I realized that I had a strained relationship with my own body, and sensual massage gave me a chance to change that. It's more about you than it is about someone else. It's an experience that teaches you to accept yourself and feel comfortable in your skin."

This idea intrigued me. Until then, I had gotten used to ignoring or criticizing my body. Every imperfection had become a reason for insecurity. Imagining an experience that would change my self-perception seemed impossible but tempting.

Ioana explained to me in more detail what sensual massage entails. She told me everything is built on consent and respect for personal boundaries. There was nothing vulgar or risky about it, just a form of therapy meant to help you reconnect with your own body.

"It's like learning to look at your body with different eyes," she said. "I began to realize that pleasure, relaxation, and connection with your own body are not things to be ashamed of. They are essential to feeling complete."

These words stayed with me for a long time. Ioana spoke of sensual massage as a profound, almost spiritual experience. It wasn't about anything superficial but about something that changes your relationship with yourself. I began to ask myself: Why do I feel so uncomfortable just hearing about it? Where does this shame come from?

After that conversation, I couldn't get what Ioana had told me out of my mind. I began to reflect on my relationship with my own body. It was true; I had always felt disconnected from him. Anything sensual, whether it was touch, pleasure, or simply accepting my body, seemed like something to avoid.

I realized I was carrying a baggage of shame I hadn't fully realized. I constantly wondered: Why is it so hard for me to accept the idea of exploring my own body? Why do I associate anything sensual with something forbidden or wrong?

The answers didn't come immediately, but the first question I asked myself was revealing: What does it mean to me to feel comfortable in my own body? I realized I didn't know the answer. It was something I had never fully experienced.

Ioana encouraged me to explore this idea without pressure. "You don't have to do anything that you don't feel is right for you," she told me. "But try to think about what it means to feel good in your skin—not for others, not to conform to social expectations, but just for you."

This suggestion was a small but essential step. I had begun to realize that many of my thoughts about my body and sensuality were not indeed mine. They had been inherited from family, society, and my early experiences. Ioana made me understand that before making any decisions about sensual massage, I needed to reevaluate my own beliefs.

As I continued to reflect, I felt caught between scepticism and curiosity. On the one hand, I wondered if I could ever try such an experience. On the other hand, I wanted to understand why Ioana was so excited. "What if sensual massage could help me get rid of this shame that has been haunting me for so many years?" I asked myself.

I wasn't ready to jump in but was prepared to explore the idea. I told myself that no matter the outcome, what mattered was allowing myself to reflect, ask questions, and take a small step outside my comfort zone.

One day, while journaling, I jotted down a simple but powerful question: What would it be like to enjoy my body without feeling ashamed? Just by asking that question, I felt an unexpected sense of relief. Maybe the answer wasn't clear yet, but for the first time, I was starting to allow myself to explore.

The conversation with Ioana didn't immediately convince me to try sensual massage, but it was the starting point for a profound transformation. It was the moment I started asking myself the right questions and realized that the shame holding me back wasn't a permanent part of me—it was just a wall that could be torn down.

Conclusion: Sensual Massage as a Pathway to Healing, Connection, and Liberation

Sensual massage is a profoundly transformative practice that holds the potential to redefine our relationship with our bodies, emotions, and connections with others. By confronting societal shame and embracing intentional touch, it paves the way for a life of greater self-awareness, emotional freedom, and meaningful intimacy. This conclusion delves into the multifaceted ways sensual massage offers healing and liberation, the societal barriers it challenges, and the broader cultural shift it can inspire.

The Healing Power of Intentional Touch

At its core, sensual massage is more than a physical act—it is a deeply emotional and psychological experience. Its benefits extend far beyond the immediate sensations of relaxation or pleasure, offering long-term effects that enhance overall well-being.

Reclaiming the Body

Shame often creates a disconnection between individuals and their bodies, fostering feelings of unworthiness, discomfort, or even disdain. Sensual massage provides a safe, judgment-free space where individuals can reconnect with their physical selves. Through mindful touch, individuals are invited to:

- **Acknowledge their physical sensations:** By focusing on the present moment, they can experience their body as a source of comfort and empowerment.

- **Celebrate their uniqueness:** Sensual massage highlights the beauty and functionality of the body, regardless of societal standards.

This reclamation of the body is particularly impactful for individuals who have experienced trauma, body-image issues, or cultural stigmas around physicality.

Emotional Release and Healing

The body often stores emotions that have not been fully processed, particularly those tied to shame, guilt, or trauma. Sensual massage allows these emotions to surface in a supportive and nurturing environment. Many participants report feelings of emotional release—whether through tears, laughter, or a profound sense of relief—signalling the unburdening of long-held pain.

Fostering Trust and Connection

The consensual and intentional nature of sensual massage fosters trust between participants, whether practiced with a partner or a professional therapist. This trust becomes the foundation for:

- **Rebuilding confidence:** For those who have struggled with boundaries or past violations, sensual massage demonstrates that touch can be safe, respectful, and healing.

- **Deepening intimacy:** Couples who engage in sensual massage often find their emotional bonds strengthened, as they learn to communicate more openly and prioritize each other's well-being.

Overcoming Societal Barriers

While sensual massage offers immense benefits, its potential is often overshadowed by societal shame and misunderstanding. Cultural taboos, misconceptions about sexuality, and rigid norms around touch contribute to the stigmatization of this practice.

Challenging Shame

Shame thrives in secrecy and societal judgment. Sensual massage directly confronts these dynamics by creating spaces for vulnerability, self-expression, and acceptance. It reminds individuals that:

- **The body is not a source of shame:** Rather, it is a vessel for pleasure, connection, and healing.

- **Sensuality is natural:** Embracing touch and sensation is an intrinsic part of the human experience, not something to be feared or condemned.

By normalizing discussions around sensual massage, society can begin to dismantle the stigma that prevents individuals from accessing its benefits.

Dispelling Misconceptions

The association of sensual massage with sexuality often leads to its misrepresentation and stigmatization. Educating the public about the therapeutic and emotional aspects of this practice is essential for reducing stigma. This involves:

- **Highlighting its healing potential:** Sensual massage is not solely about arousal but about fostering relaxation, mindfulness, and connection.

- **Reframing touch:** By emphasizing the non-sexual elements of sensual massage, society can better understand its broader applications and benefits.

A Cultural Shift Toward Acceptance

Sensual massage has the potential to inspire a broader cultural shift in how we view touch, sensuality, and the body. As more people embrace this practice, it can become a catalyst for positive change at both individual and societal levels.

Creating Safe Spaces for Vulnerability

Vulnerability is essential for personal growth and emotional healing. Sensual massage provides a framework for exploring this vulnerability in a controlled and supportive environment. These spaces can:

- **Encourage open dialogue:** Participants are invited to communicate their needs, boundaries, and fears without judgment.

- **Promote inclusivity:** Sensual massage can be practiced by individuals of all genders, ages, and relationship statuses, fostering a sense of universality and acceptance.

Shifting Attitudes Toward Sensuality

A culture that embraces sensuality as a natural and empowering part of life can counteract the shame and stigma that often surround touch and intimacy. This shift requires:

- **Education:** Providing accurate information about sensual massage through workshops, articles, and media representation.

- **Advocacy:** Highlighting stories of transformation to showcase the practice's healing potential.

- **Representation:** Ensuring that diverse bodies, identities, and experiences are visible in discussions about sensual massage.

The Role of Sensual Massage in Relationships

Sensual massage is a powerful tool for fostering connection and intimacy in relationships. By prioritizing intentional touch, couples can strengthen their emotional and physical bonds.

Building Trust

Trust is the foundation of any healthy relationship, and sensual massage offers a tangible way to build and maintain it. Through clear communication and mutual respect, partners can:

- **Explore vulnerability together:** Sharing the experience of sensual massage encourages openness and honesty.

- **Demonstrate care and consideration:** The act of giving and receiving touch reinforces the importance of mutual support.

Enhancing Intimacy

Incorporating sensual massage into a relationship can rekindle passion and deepen connection. It allows couples to:

- **Rediscover each other:** By focusing on touch and sensation, partners can reconnect on a physical and emotional level.

- **Prioritize quality time:** Sensual massage creates an opportunity to slow down and be present with one another.

Practical Steps for Embracing Sensual Massage

For those interested in exploring sensual massage, taking practical steps can make the journey accessible and rewarding.

1. Start with Self-Massage

Self-massage is an excellent way to become comfortable with touch and develop a deeper connection with your body. Techniques like using oils, focusing on areas of tension, and practicing mindfulness can help foster self-acceptance.

2. Communicate with Partners

If exploring sensual massage with a partner, open communication is essential. Discuss boundaries, desires, and intentions to ensure a positive and respectful experience.

3. Seek Professional Guidance

For those dealing with significant shame or trauma, working with a certified sensual massage therapist or somatic healer can provide a safe and supportive environment for healing.

The Broader Implications of Sensual Massage

Sensual massage is not just a personal practice—it has implications for broader societal change. By embracing its principles, we can:

- **Foster empathy:** Learning to honour and respect others' boundaries can create more compassionate relationships.

- **Normalize vulnerability:** Encouraging openness and honesty can reduce stigma around emotions and touch.

- **Promote wellness:** Sensual massage is a holistic approach to mental, physical, and emotional health, aligning with broader trends in wellness culture.

A Vision for the Future

Imagine a world where sensuality is celebrated rather than shamed, where individuals feel empowered to connect with their bodies and each other without fear of judgment. Sensual massage has the potential to bring us closer to this vision by promoting trust, acceptance, and emotional freedom.

By creating spaces for vulnerability, fostering connection, and challenging societal norms, sensual massage can inspire a cultural shift toward greater openness and compassion. It reminds us that the body is not a source of shame but a vessel for healing, pleasure, and profound human connection.

Final Thoughts

Sensual massage offers a powerful pathway to healing, connection, and liberation. Its emphasis on intentional touch and mindfulness provides individuals with the tools to confront shame, embrace vulnerability, and foster deeper relationships. Despite societal barriers, the transformative potential of sensual massage cannot be overstated—it is a practice that celebrates the body's innate wisdom and beauty.

As we work to normalize sensual massage and reduce stigma, we move closer to a world where touch is seen not as taboo, but as a fundamental part of the human experience. By embracing this practice, individuals and communities alike can rediscover the profound healing power of connection, trust, and self-acceptance.

ABOUT THE AUTHOR

Alaric James Northcott is the author of *The Eternity*, a contemplative work that delves into the journey of self-discovery and spiritual enlightenment. In this book, Northcott shares his personal quest to understand the concept of eternity, exploring themes of meditation, prayer, and introspection. He reflects on overcoming challenges, such as confronting disruptive spiritual influences, and emphasizes the importance of forgiveness and love in achieving inner peace. Through his narrative, Northcott invites readers to embark on their own spiritual journeys, encouraging a deeper connection with the divine and a rediscovery of the bonds that unite all of existence.

The Eternity was independently published on November 18, 2023, and is available in paperback.

Amazon UK

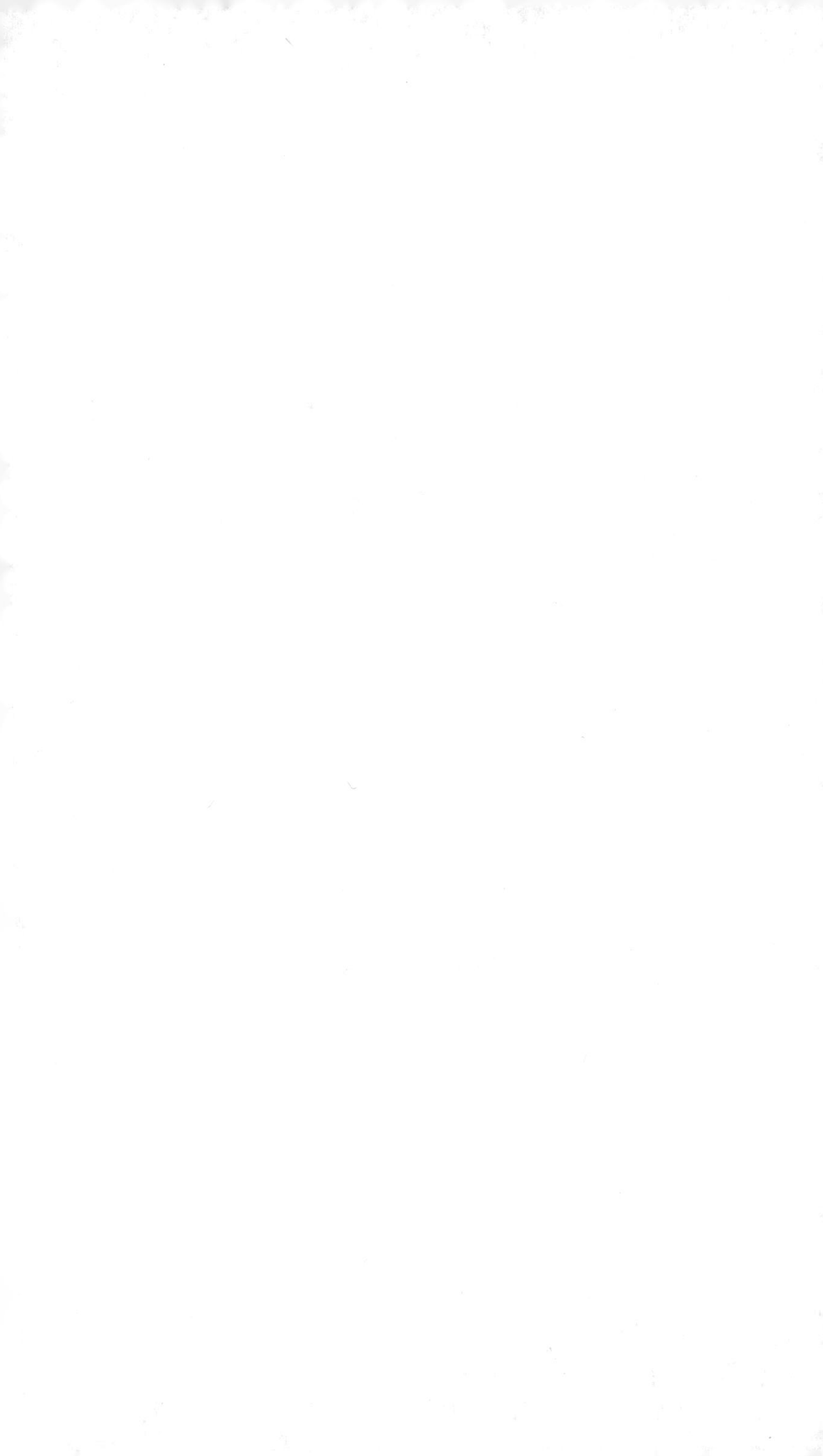